A LITTLE BOOK OF SELF CARE

AROMATHERAPY

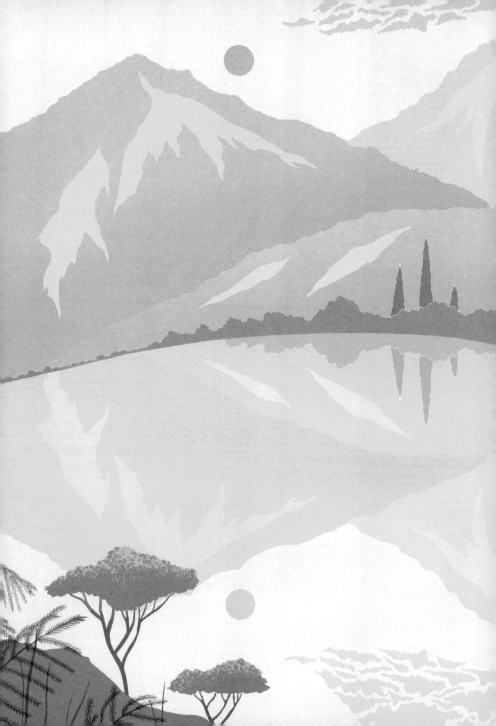

DK

A LITTLE BOOK OF SELF CARE

AROMATHERAPY

HARNESS THE POWER OF ESSENTIAL OILS TO RELAX, RESTORE, AND REVITALIZE

LOUISE ROBINSON

DK | Penguin Random House

Editor Ian Fitzgerald
Designer Natalie Clay
Senior Editor Rona Skene
Project Art Editor Louise Brigenshaw
Editorial Assistant Kiron Gill
Jacket Designer Amy Cox
Jackets Coordinator Lucy Philpott
Senior Production Editor Tony Phipps
Production Controller Rebecca Parton
Creative Technical Support Sonia Charbonnier
Managing Editor Dawn Henderson
Managing Art Editor Marianne Markham
Art Director Maxine Pedliham
Publishing Director Mary-Clare Jerram

Illustrated by Harriet Lee-Merrion

First published in Great Britain in 2020 by
Dorling Kindersley Limited
DK, One Embassy Gardens, 8 Viaduct Gardens,
London, SW11 7BW

10 9 8 7 6 5 4 3 2 1
001–318951–Dec/2020

DISCLAIMER see page 144

A CIP catalogue record for this book is available from the British Library.
ISBN: 978-0-2414-4366-8

Printed and bound in China

For the curious
www.dk.com

MIX
Paper from responsible sources
FSC www.fsc.org FSC™ C018179

This book was made with Forest Stewardship Council ™ certified paper – one small step in DK's commitment to a sustainable future. For more information go to www.dk.com/our-green-pledge

CONTENTS

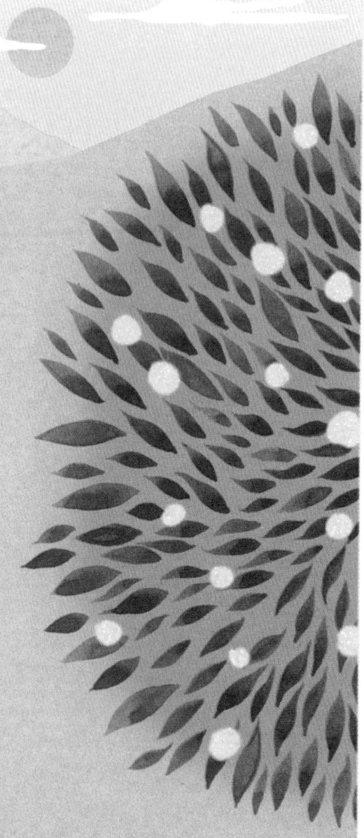

FOREWORD

I have always been fascinated by fragrance. As a little girl, I was enchanted by the heady, sweet scent of roses in our family garden, collecting their petals and spending hours trying to recreate their perfume. Even now, whenever I smell a rose my mind returns to those childhood flowers. So it's no surprise as an adult I was drawn to aromatherapy, especially as a busy working mum with three young sons. I found that using essential oils helped me to cope, and eventually I decided it was something I wanted to use to help other people in their lives, too. After training with Neal's Yard Remedies in London, I gave up my corporate career and became a therapist.

Working in my practice and within the NHS in the area of mental health, I still marvel at the profound power of aromatherapy to transform a person's health or spirit. My main focus at work is on using essential oils in massage therapy, where the healing power of touch, the mood-altering aromas, and the oils' therapeutic compounds combine holistically to improve my clients' physical, mental, and emotional conditions.

In this book, I want to show you that aromatherapy is not just taking in pleasing aromas to make you feel happy (though it certainly is that) – it also encompasses relaxing and healing massage, skin-repairing and first-aid remedies, practices to balance your body's rhythms, blends for boosting immunity and so much more.

The book begins by explaining what aromatherapy and essential oils are, then how to use oils correctly, safely, and beneficially. After that, it explores the ways that essential oils can be used. Finally, there are the remedies, blends, and rituals especially created for this book and for you to use yourself, at home. They are divided into "Wellbeing" treatments, which give you that extra lift in mind, body, and spirit that we all need from time to time, and "Healing" treatments designed to address, relieve, and help cure a range of conditions.

Being holistic, aromatherapy's benefits always go beyond the issue you are treating: if you're using essential oils to calm a rash or soothe aching muscles, you will also emerge from the experience feeling calmer, happier, more balanced, or energized. It's what makes aromatherapy so special and so powerful. My hope is that this book will inspire you to use that power from now on, simply and effectively, and make it a part of your self-care routine.

Writing this book has been a joy and a privilege for me, and I truly hope that you find it helpful and useful in the aromatic journey that lies ahead of you.

Louise Robinson

GETTING STARTED

WHAT IS AROMATHERAPY?

A practice with origins in ancient history, aromatherapy has never been more relevant than it is today, when so many of us are taking a more natural and holistic approach to health and wellbeing.

ANCIENT ORIGINS

For millennia, plants were our only form of medicine, and our ancestors in ancient Egypt, Greece, and Rome used aromatherapy-style remedies both for healing and in religious ceremonies. Modern aromatherapy began in the 1930s, pioneered in France by chemist René-Maurice Gattefossé and military surgeon Jean Valnet, and in Austria by beautician and biochemist Marguerite Maury.

A NATURAL PRACTICE

Building on the work of these early pioneers, aromatherapy developed from the second half of the twentieth century into the therapeutic use of highly concentrated and powerful essential oils extracted from aromatic plants to heal the body and mind and to promote wellness. As its name suggests, this takes place largely through the inhalation of essential oil aromas, but also through the application of essential oils to the skin (see pages 16–17).

AN ALL-ROUND THERAPY

On its own or as part of practices such as massage, meditation, yoga, and mindfulness, aromatherapy is the ideal antidote to the stresses of modern life. Easy to use and incorporate into a daily self-care routine, aromatherapy can promote wellbeing, relieve symptoms, and heal the body and mind. It can also provide relief and support for those undergoing medical treatment.

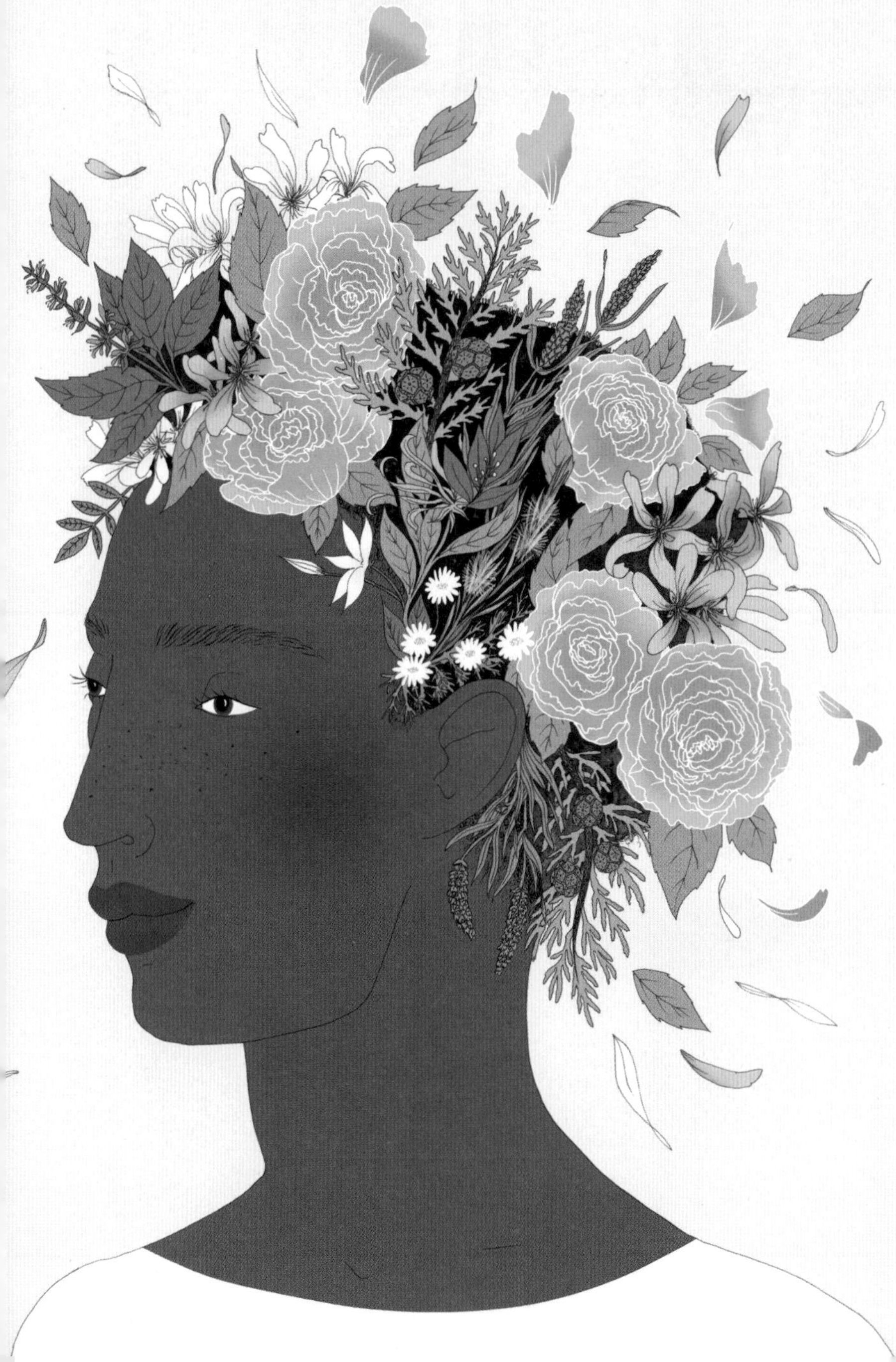

BENEFITS OF AROMATHERAPY

Aromatherapy is both holistic and specific: it acts on the mind, body, and spirit to treat the entire person, but can also be used to "target" specific ailments and conditions. It's a simple practice, too, and once you begin using essential oils you'll be able to feel the benefits straight away. If you are feeling anxious, for example, inhaling soothing bergamot will begin to calm you down immediately. In the longer term, essential oil-based treatments for ongoing conditions such as joint or muscle pain, migraines, or respiratory illness can help to alleviate symptoms.

AIDS DIGESTION
Antispasmodic peppermint relaxes muscles and loosens the bowels. Like cardamom, it is also an analgesic, so both oils will help ease pain and discomfort.

BALANCES HORMONES
Sweet fennel can help with menopausal symptoms where oestrogen is fluctuating, while geranium, rose, and cypress alleviate symptoms caused by hormonal imbalances.

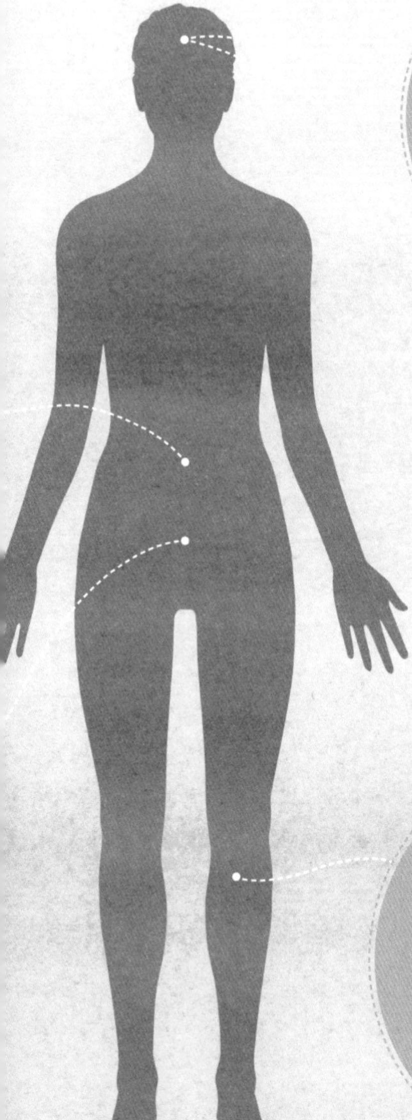

GIVES FOCUS
Essential oil aromas stimulate the limbic brain, which controls concentration and alertness. Rosemary is particularly effective.

CALMS AND RELAXES
Ester-rich compounds in oils such as clary sage, lavender, and bergamot cause the brain to release GABA, an anti-anxiety and sleep-friendly neurotransmitter.

HELPS YOU HEAL
The anti-inflammatory and antiseptic properties of many oils ease pain, repair injuries, fight infections, and boost immunity. Juniper and lemon flush out toxins and improve blood flow.

WHAT ARE ESSENTIAL OILS?

Essential oils are highly concentrated liquids, rich in natural chemical compounds, carefully extracted from aromatic plants. In aromatherapy they are used in various ways to heal and promote wellness.

WHERE DO THEY COME FROM?
We extract essential oils from just a few natural sources: the leaves, petals, stems, and roots of plants and flowers; dried and fresh seeds; the skins and rinds of citrus fruits; and tree resins and barks.

Research indicates that plants create oils mostly as a defence against animals and insects (which gives them their antiseptic, "medical" properties), and to attract pollinators (which partly explains their pleasant aromas).

HOW ARE OILS EXTRACTED?
Distillation is the most common way of harvesting essential oils. Plant parts are heated in a chamber and the resulting vapour is cooled and condensed into a highly concentrated liquid "essence".

Another method, used especially on fruit rinds, is expression. Oil is squeezed from the fruit by putting it under intense pressure. Recently, experts have developed a method, using carbon dioxide, of gathering the essence of delicate items such as flower petals.

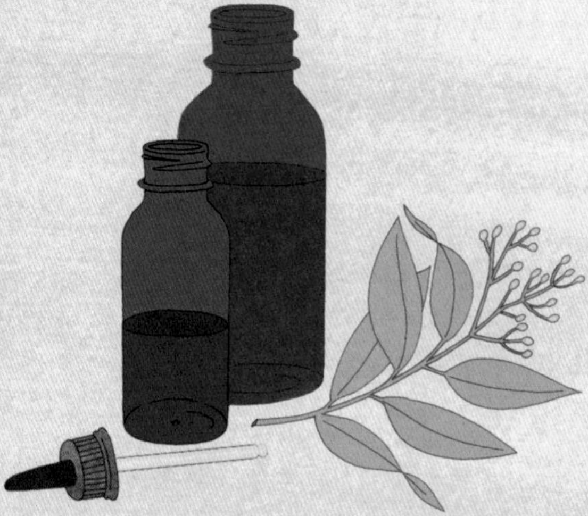

WHAT'S IN ESSENTIAL OILS?

Each of the around 150 essential oils in use today is made up of about 100 chemical compounds, and every oil has its own profile, with some compounds more dominant than others. Tea tree, for example, is rich in healing antiseptic and antibacterial elements, while bergamot contains more calming components. It is this mix of compounds in their differing proportions that gives each oil its own aroma and therapeutic properties.

WHY DO WE BLEND THEM?

Finding the right balance between healing and calming essential oils is one of the main reasons we blend them. Plus, all oils also contain tiny traces of other chemicals that also have beneficial effects on the mind and body, and it's often in their interaction with other compounds that the magic of aromatherapy happens. Experimenting with combinations of oils gives you untold opportunities to create blends to suit your unique needs.

HOW ESSENTIAL OILS WORK

Essential oils work on our bodies in two ways – as aromas targeting the brain and the lungs, and as liquid that heals the skin before being absorbed into our blood and lymph circulatory systems to work from within.

There's some complex chemistry at work in aromatherapy, but at a basic level essential oils work to heal mind and body, and promote balance between them. Around 150 essential oils are used in aromatherapy, each with its own unique therapeutic properties: chamomile, for example, is balancing and calming, while tea tree is an excellent antiseptic, and thyme will help with pain relief.

Because aromatherapy is holistic, it benefits the whole person, in addition to any specific treatment an oil is used for. Frankincense, for instance, is used to treat backache, due to its effectiveness as a painkiller. But frankincense also contains calming and stabilizing aromatic compounds that help settle anxiety – and this will also play a part in further relieving the user's back issues.

Essential oils start to work as soon as you inhale their aromas, and go on working after they are absorbed by your skin. From there, they work on the brain, lungs, bloodstream, and lymphatic system in deeply beneficial ways (see opposite).

THE BRAIN

Essential oils act on the brain's limbic system, the emotional centre that controls mood-altering hormones and neurochemicals. The linalool compounds in lavender, for example, regulate pleasure-giving dopamine and cut adrenaline, reducing anxiety.

THE LUNGS

When we breathe in essential oils, molecules travel into the lungs, and from there they enter the bloodstream. They also pass into the lymphatic system, where they can flush out toxins and boost the immune system.

THE BLOODSTREAM

Oils applied to the skin are absorbed through the pores, where their compounds enter the bloodstream and are carried round the body.

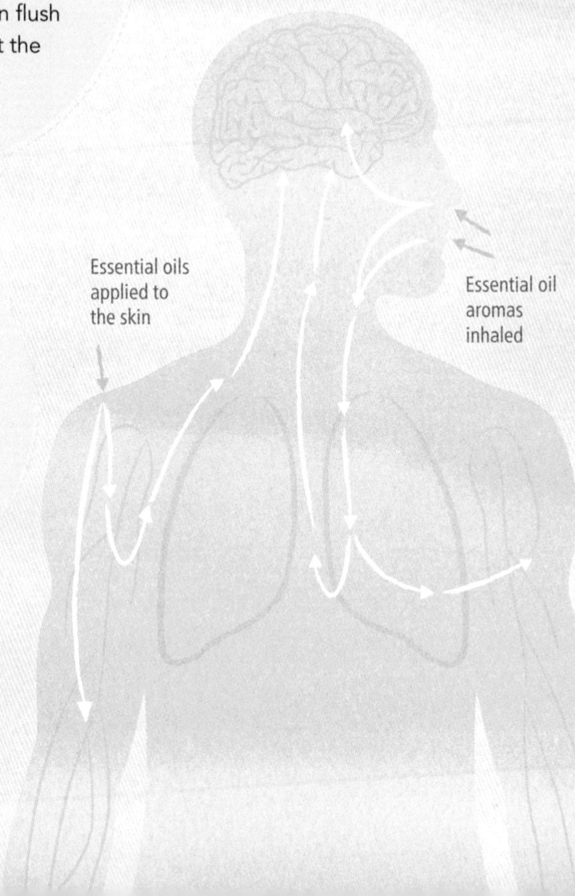

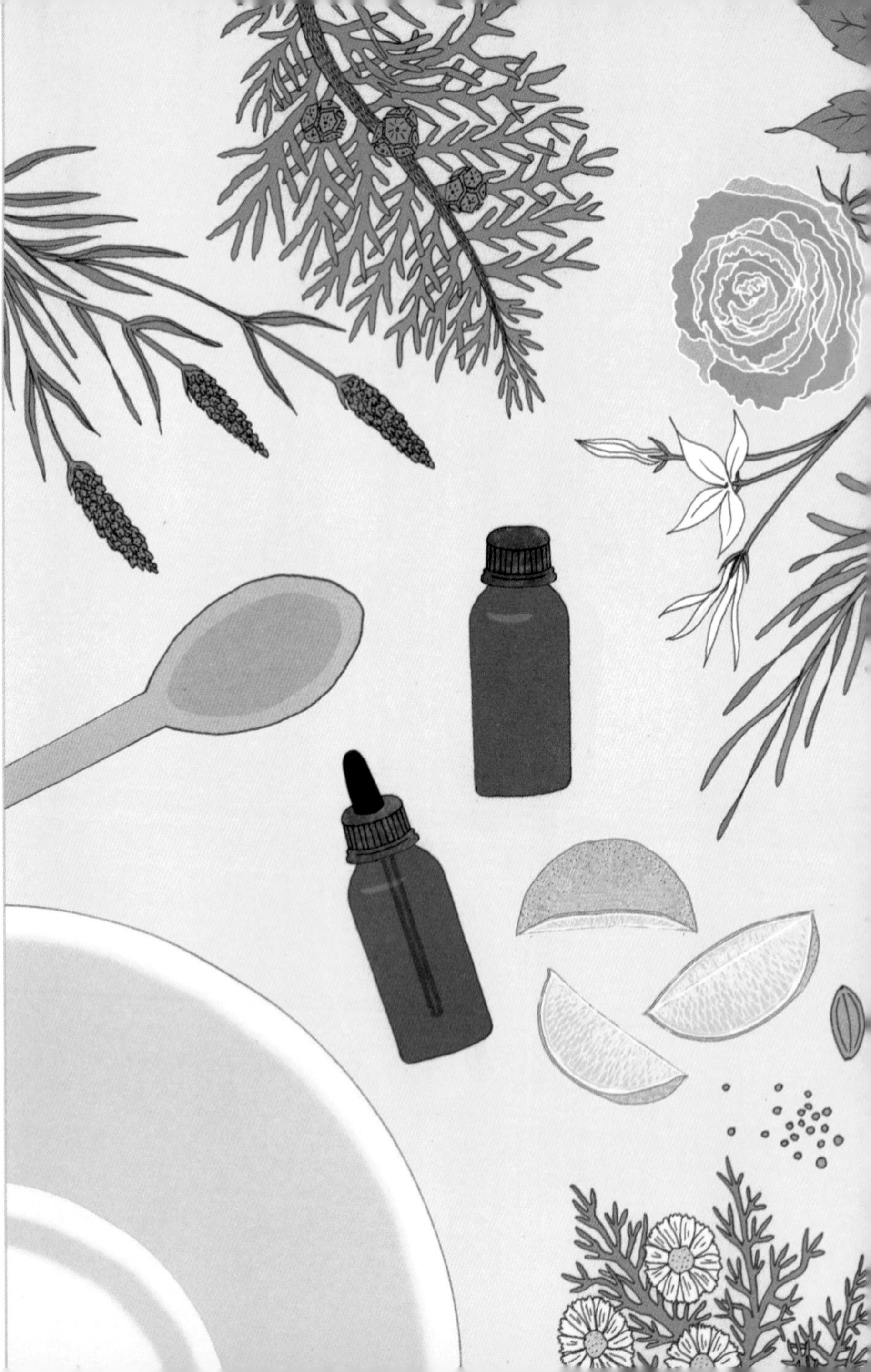

CREATING YOUR OWN BLENDS

When you combine essential oils something special happens, an alchemy that allows you to create blends tailored to your unique needs. It's an easy and enjoyable process – and the more you practise, the more confident you'll become at blending.

BEFORE YOU BEGIN

Consider what the blend is for, and how you'll use it: is it for inhaling, or to use on your skin? Maybe it's both. If so, what form should the blend take: bath or shower oil, cream, lotion, gel, or balm?

Do you need anything else, such as base oils or items of equipment, such as jars or bottles?

Check the oils' safety and allergy information.

Choose oils you like. You'll use the blend more if you love its aroma.

Use the dilution table on pages 22–23 to calculate how much essential oil and carrier liquid to use.

BLENDING GUIDELINES

When you are starting out, blend a maximum of three oils. For balance, use oils with light top notes, such as lemon; floral middle notes, like geranium; and rich base notes, like sandalwood.

Less is more: use just one or two drops to start. Essential oils are powerful; a single drop of a strong oil can transform a blend.

If you make a mistake, just start again. Adding more oils to a "bad" blend only makes it worse.

Keep a record of ingredients and amounts used so that you can recreate successful blends.

INGREDIENTS AND EQUIPMENT

Essential oils are not the only equipment you'll need when you begin your blending journey. These are the items you should have when you put together an aromatherapy kit.

As you begin your aromatherapy self-care experience you'll need some added ingredients to help you to create your own face, body, and wellbeing products. Having the right equipment ensures you can make and store your creations safely.

NATURAL INGREDIENTS

These can be combined with essential oils either to create a base or carrier for your oil blend, or for therapeutic use.

Base oils form the basis of your aromatherapy face and body creams and lotions, as well as your bath and shower blends. They are a vital component of any blend, as essential oils are very powerful and must always be diluted. Use plant oils such as grapeseed or almond oil, which are low-odour and easily absorbed by the skin. Where possible, they should be organic, additive-free, and unfragranced.

For therapeutic use, you can blend essential oils with other healing ingredients such as aloe vera gel, or shea butter, coconut oil, and beeswax for making balms. Add Epsom salts and oats to an essential oil-infused bath to soothe sore muscles or soften the skin. Diluting

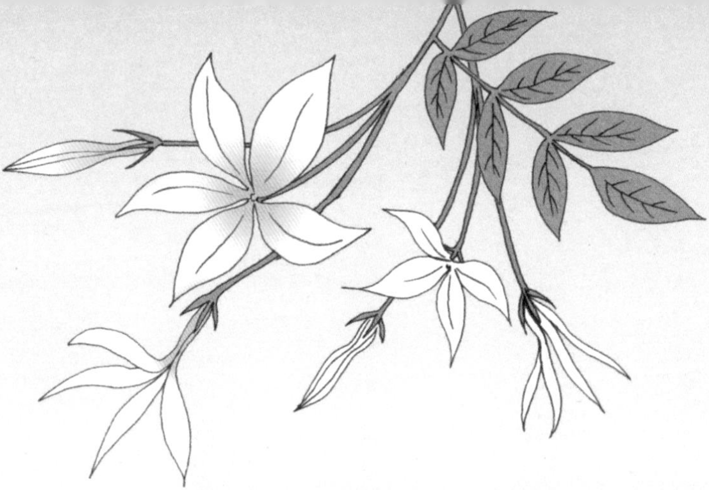

essential oils with rose water or orange flower water will create a spritz – an aromatic water, which cools and calms the skin instantly.

EQUIPMENT

Glass, aluminium, and plastic jars and bottles. These should be dark in colour to protect your blends from sunlight, which can degrade an oil's properties.
Oil storage case (optional) as extra protection against sunlight.
Tissues for inhalation.
Small plastic bags to carry tissues.
Aromasticks (see pages 44–45) for inhalation.
Room diffuser (see pages 48–49).
Small rollette bottles (see pages 38–39) to apply oil blends to the skin.
Mixing stick, glass if possible, as it is easier to clean and keep sterile.
Glass or metal bowls, for mixing blends.
Flannels and towels, for compresses and steam inhalation treatments.
Muslin squares, around 20x20cm (8x8in), to make oil-infused bath "parcels".
Foot bowl or a flat-bottomed washing-up bowl.

USING ESSENTIAL OILS SAFELY

Although very powerful, essential oils represent little or no risk when used correctly – and always in dilution. Follow the guidance here on handling oils for an enjoyable and safe aromatherapy experience.

TAKE A PATCH TEST

It's important when using any oil for the first time to perform a patch test, especially if you have sensitive skin or a skin condition such as eczema. This test is a simple and safe way to determine if your skin is allergic by placing a tiny dab of an oil on the body to see if there is any reaction. Be aware that patch testing is not 100 per cent accurate as not all reactions to oils show on the skin, so you should also check the list on pages 136–138 before you use a new oil.

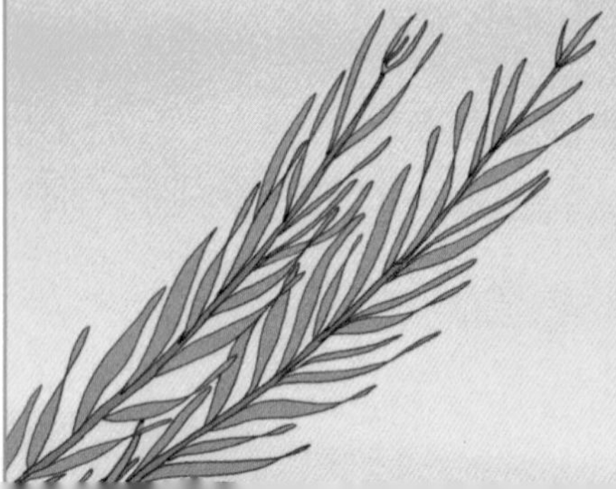

01

Selecting an essential oil of your choice and an unfragranced skin cream, make up a 10ml "normal" dilution (see table opposite).

02

Apply a small amount to your inner elbow and leave for 24 hours. If you experience any irritation, swelling, or discomfort, wash off the dilution straight away.

03

If, at the end of the 24-hour test period, there is no redness or irritation, you can safely apply the oil to a larger area of your body.

ESSENTIAL OIL KNOW-HOW

Never ingest essential oils, as they can be toxic, and do not apply them neat to the skin. If undiluted oil gets on the skin, coat the area in vegetable oil then wash it off. If it gets in your eyes, rinse with cold water immediately and seek medical advice.

Keep essential oils out of reach of children. The blends in this book have been formulated specifically for adults, so are not suitable for children.

If you are trying for a baby, breastfeeding, or have an ongoing medical condition, check pages 136–138 for guidance on using specific essential oils. If you have a nut allergy, check the ingredients of your base oil before use.

DILUTION TABLE

Essential oils must be diluted before using them on skin: blends can be made up in different strengths, according to their intended use. There are three dilution strengths: the weakest for sensitive skin and conditions such as pregnancy, the "standard" dilution for normal skin and body blends, and the strongest for therapeutic applications and in bath oils. This table sets out the maximum quantities of essential oils to use with different amounts of base oil.

AMOUNT OF BASE INGREDIENT (eg, oil, cream, gel)	**10ml (0.35fl oz)**	**20ml (0.70fl oz)**	**30ml (1fl oz)**
Delicate skin; facial massage; trying to conceive; pregnancy; breastfeeding; suffering ill health	2 drops	4 drops	6 drops
Body massage blends for non-sensitive skin	5 drops	10 drops	15 drops
Therapeutic blends; bath oils	10 drops	20 drops	30 drops

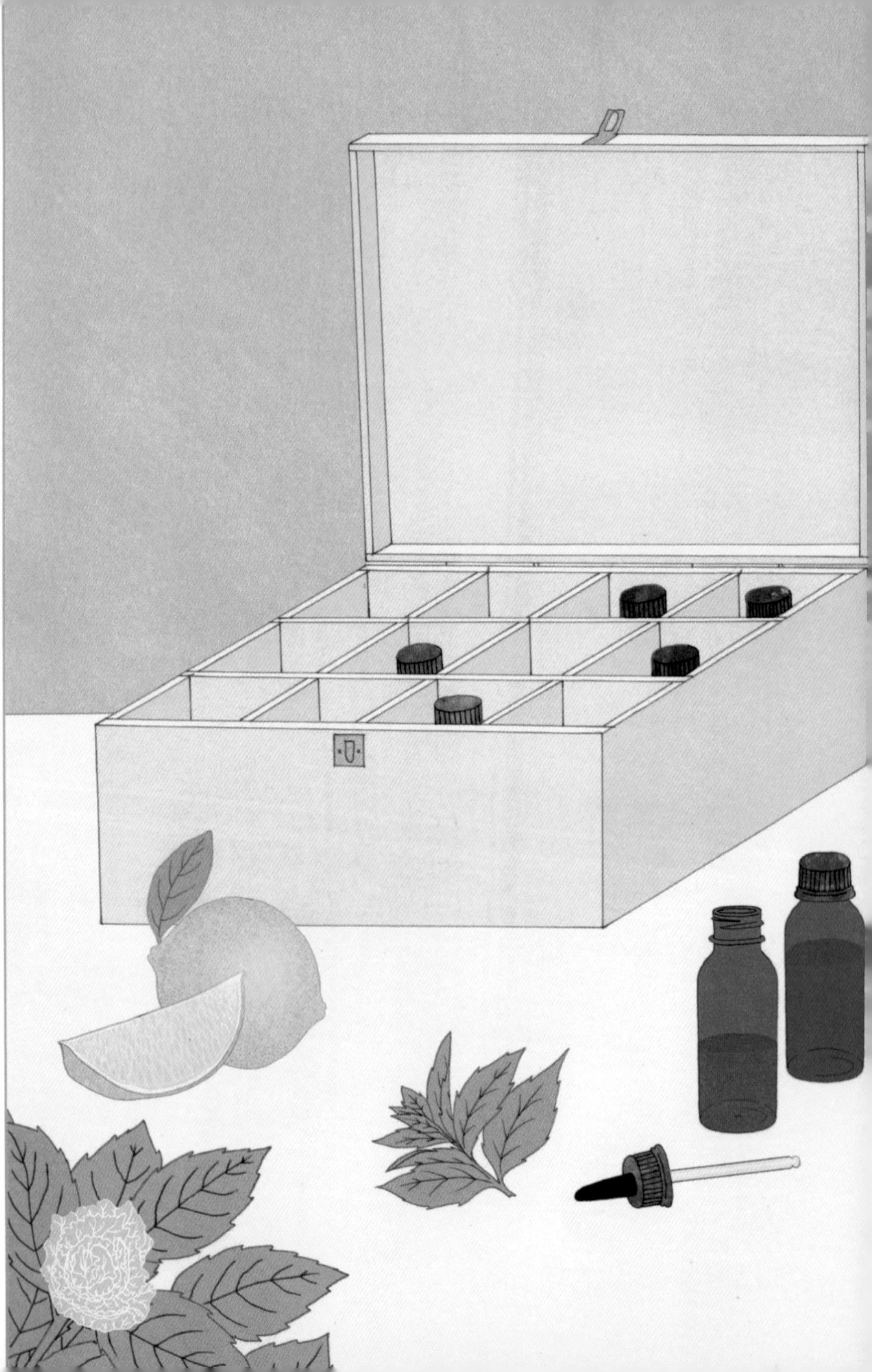

BUYING AND STORING ESSENTIAL OILS

Now that you are at the start of an exciting journey into the world of aromatherapy, it's worth taking note of this advice on buying and storing your oils to help you make the most of their healing properties.

You don't need to spend a lot on a huge array of oils: start small, see what you like and find most useful, and add to your collection when you know your preferences.

The four most commonly used oils are geranium, Roman chamomile, tea tree, and lavender. Use them to form the basis of your collection.

Buy organic oils as these have not been contaminated with synthetic fertilizers and have a high therapeutic action.

Always purchase pure oils, with no added ingredients.

Don't buy oils that have been stored or displayed in sunlight, as this may have caused deterioration in their quality; once you buy, store them in a cool place and out of direct sunlight.

Check the botanical name, which is in Latin, on the bottle. If no Latin name is shown it may mean that the oil contains additives or has been adulterated in some other way – do not buy these. See pages 136–138 for a full list of all the oils suggested in this book, with their botanical names.

Buy small quantities of essential oils regularly. Shelf life varies between six months and two years – check the bottle when you buy.

USING ESSENTIAL OILS

SKIN APPLICATIONS

Not only are skin treatments an effective way to get essential oil compounds into the body, but application methods such as massage and bathing can be joyful and mood-enhancing in themselves. And, of course, you also get to breathe in those life-affirming aromas as the oils work on your skin.

UNDERSTANDING MASSAGE OILS

Using essential oils with massage is a perfect therapeutic combination: the power of touch and scent merging together to enhance each other's healing properties for a wide range of physical and emotional conditions.

Massage has become one of the most popular ways to experience aromatherapy. Whether you try self-massage or place yourself in the hands of an aromatherapy practitioner, you'll find it extremely beneficial – and addictive!

WHY USE MASSAGE?

Massage with essential oils delivers a threefold benefit. Before you even begin, the oils' aromas will activate receptors in the brain to "tell" you how to feel. Depending on the oil, you may begin to feel calmer, more energized, or joyful.

Next, massage is therapeutic. It relieves stress, eases tension, and can help with muscle and joint complaints. Self-massage is also deeply comforting, a profound act of self-care only you can administer.

Finally, as the essential oils are absorbed by the skin, they relieve and repair damaged muscles and tissues, then enter the bloodstream and the lymphatic system to improve your circulation and remove impurities.

There are, however, some circumstances in which massage may be unhelpful – for instance if you have a thrombosis, a fever, or feel unwell. Never massage open wounds or broken skin, and avoid broken bones, bruises, and arthritic swelling. Always make up massage blends using the appropriate base oils (see pages 20–21).

BODY AND FACE BLENDS

Massage oils are usually made in one of two strengths, depending on whether they are for use on the body or the face.

Body blends have a relatively high concentration of essential oils within the base oil, as the body's skin is more robust than that of the face.

Face blends are less concentrated, so as not to irritate the more sensitive facial skin. See pages 22–23 for more on diluting oils.

WARM AND COLD COMPRESSES

A compress infused with therapeutic essential oils is an effective way to treat specific areas of the body, especially when they are too painful or sensitive for massage. Use a warm or cold compress, depending on the issue you want to treat.

Compresses can be used to treat a variety of issues (see right), but it's best to avoid using them on babies or elderly people, as their bodies are less able to deal with sudden temperature changes.

WARM COMPRESSES

A warm compress is a cloth or flannel soaked in tepid-to-warm water infused with healing essential oils. When you place the oil-infused cloth on the affected area of the body, the gentle heat and mild pressure opens up blood vessels and improves circulation. This allows the oils to enter the body and deliver their therapeutic benefits. Leave the compress in place for around a minute or until it cools. If necessary, create a new warm water infusion and repeat the compression once or twice more.

COLD COMPRESSES

Soothing, pain-relieving compresses soaked in cold water and essential oils are simple first-aid remedies for a range of skin complaints. They also reduce swelling as they cause blood vessels to constrict, reducing blood flow. To use, soak a cloth or flannel in cold water infused with essential oil. Wring out excess water and place the cloth directly onto the affected areas for 2–3 minutes. Repeat if necessary.

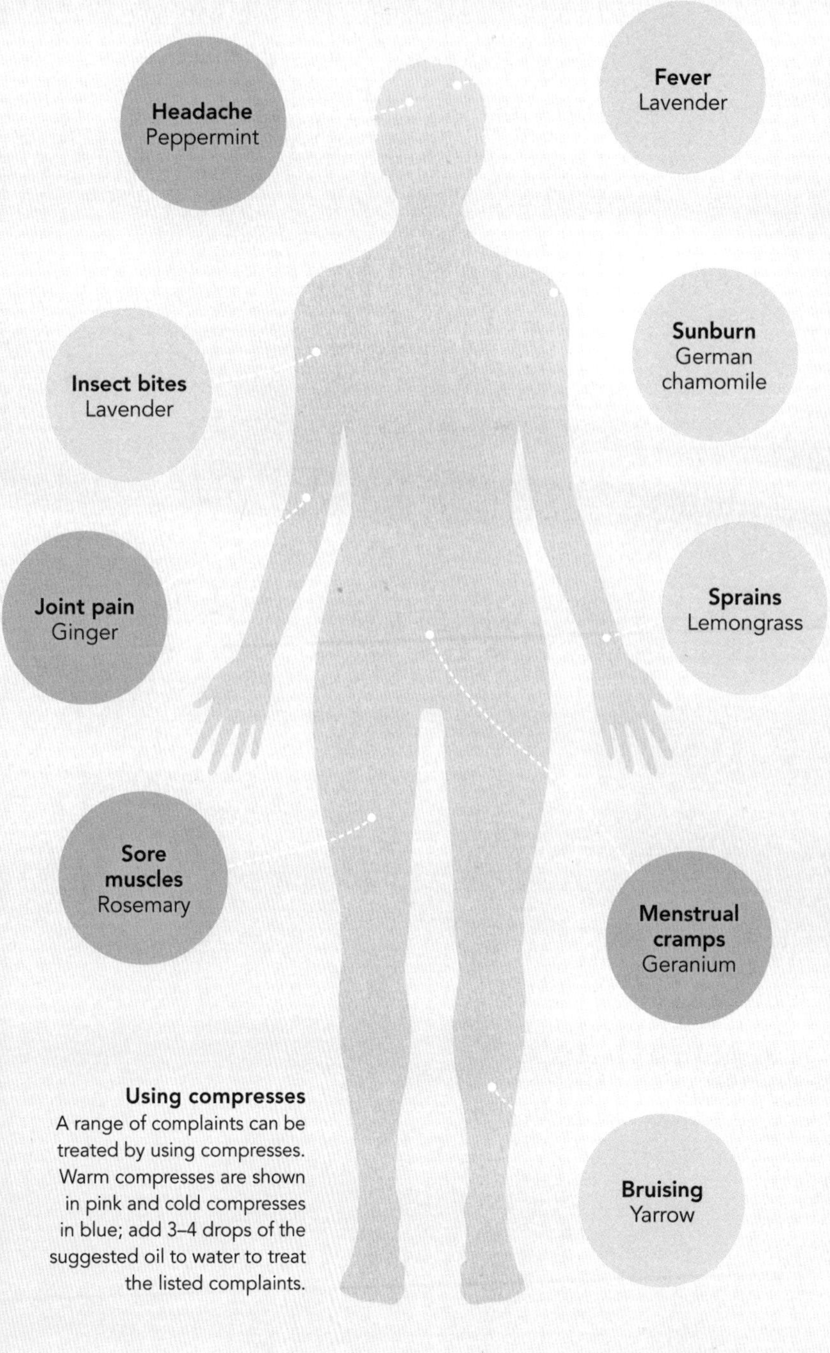

Using compresses
A range of complaints can be treated by using compresses. Warm compresses are shown in pink and cold compresses in blue; add 3–4 drops of the suggested oil to water to treat the listed complaints.

USING CREAMS, LOTIONS, AND GELS

Using oils in a creamy base is an excellent way to deliver their healing benefits, and to nourish the skin. You can add ingredients to boost their effectiveness, and make essential oil creams part of your daily skin-care routine.

Creams, lotions, and gels combine well with essential oils to make aromatherapy blends that can be used to help with a range of skin issues or as part of your skin-care regime.

CREAM AND LOTION BASES

Creams and lotions are a mix of water, which makes them easily absorbable, and glycerin and plant oils, which moisturize and soothe the skin. Essential oils are added to a cream or lotion base – see pages 22–23 for advice on the proportions to use for body and facial blends. Always use organic, unfragranced creams and lotions, free of artificial additives, so as not to affect the efficacy of the essential oils you have chosen.

Creams usually contain more plant oils than lotions, making them thicker and more nourishing, and better suited to treat acne, sunburn, or other conditions where a "barrier" is required. Lotions work better where essential oils need to be absorbed into the skin quickly, such as helping with sore muscles or verrucas. To re-use empty cream jars, boil them in a large pan for five minutes and leave them to dry naturally before refilling them.

SUPPLEMENTING BLENDS

Blends of creams or lotions and essential oils can be enhanced by adding in an extra 10 per cent of health-enriching plant oils such as wheatgerm, avocado, or argan oil. All are rich in cell-regenerating antioxidants, vitamins, minerals, and essential fatty acids, helping to repair, replenish, and rejuvenate the skin.

WHEN TO USE GELS

Thick, cooling gels are a good alternative to creams and lotions. They are ideal for treating irritated or inflamed skin, or for first-aid use on cuts and grazes. Cooling aloe vera makes an excellent base for a skin-healing gel.

MAKING BALMS

Homemade balms have been used for centuries to heal dry, damaged, and fragile skin, while moisturizing and adding fragrance. A little pot of balm is a supercharged remedy for a range of issues, including cracked, dry lips and sunburn.

Balms are solidified oils mixed with butters and waxes, which gives them a thicker consistency than water-based oils and creams. They "sit" on the skin for longer, which makes them ideal for use as salves, skin cleansers, solid perfumes, face masks, moisturizers, and even a tamer for unruly eyebrows. They will also treat dry skin, chafing, damaged cuticles, and sore, hurt feet.

MAKE YOUR OWN BALM

This recipe uses almond oil as its base, but you can also use sunflower oil or grapeseed oil for a lighter balm. Wheatgerm oil is nourishing, and macerated calendula oil is excellent for healing wounds. Lavender is good for all-round use in balms, but you can use other oils to suit your needs.

Makes 30g (1fl oz)

Essential oils:

- 6 drops of lavender

Other items:

1 tsp of beeswax pellets; 1 tsp of shea butter; 1 tbsp of almond oil; small saucepan; heatproof glass bowl; mixing stick; glass jar with lid

How to make

Half-fill the saucepan with water and place on a low heat. Put the glass bowl on the saucepan and add all the ingredients, except the essential oil, allowing them to melt. Add the essential oil to the jar, then pour in the melted ingredients. Stir the balm, then leave to cool and set.

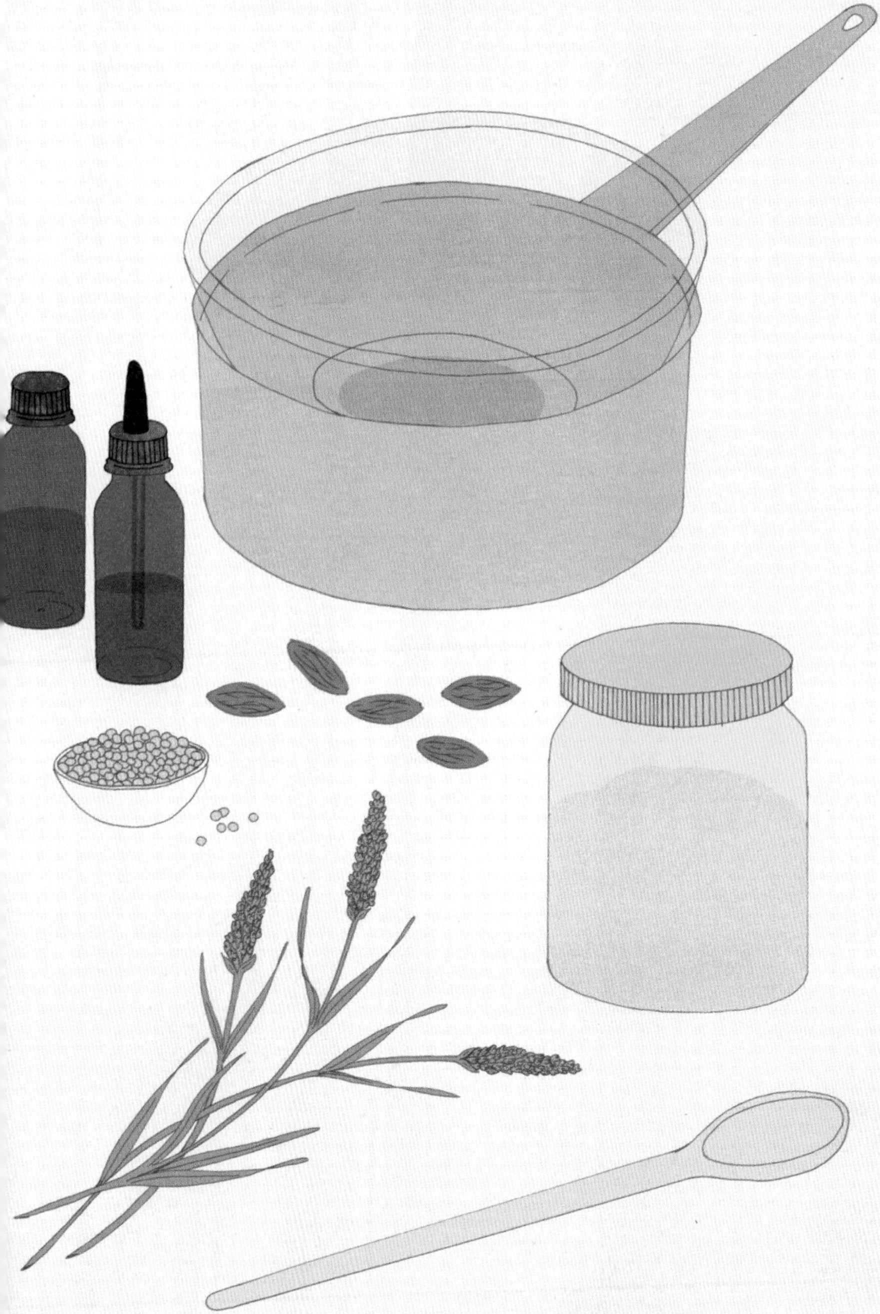

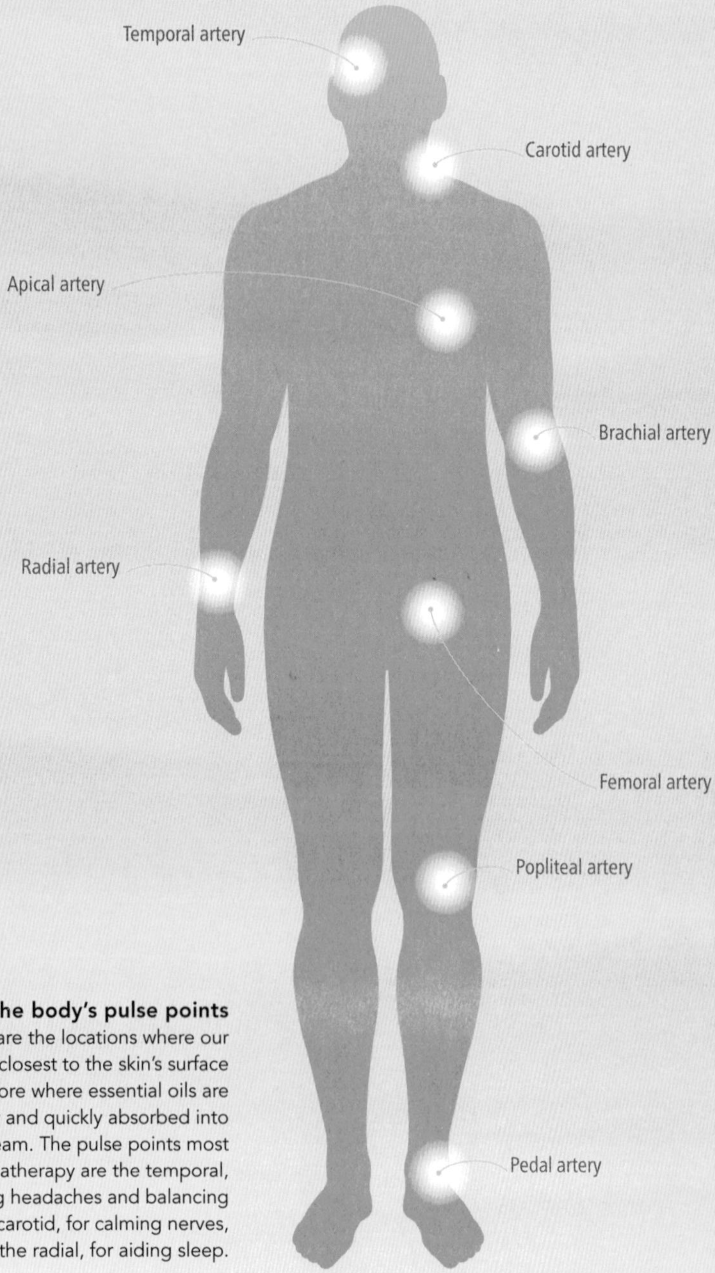

The body's pulse points

Pulse points are the locations where our arteries are closest to the skin's surface – and therefore where essential oils are most easily and quickly absorbed into the bloodstream. The pulse points most used in aromatherapy are the temporal, for relieving headaches and balancing the mind, the carotid, for calming nerves, and the radial, for aiding sleep.

USING ROLLETTES ON PULSE POINTS

The perfect pick-me-up for when you're out and about, a quick dab on your pulse points with a pocket-sized rollette and a few deep breaths deliver an instant burst of revitalizing aromas.

A rollette is a small bottle around the same size and shape as a lipstick, topped with a rollerball similar to that on a roll-on deodorant. The rollerball can be screwed on and off, allowing the bottle to be refilled.

To use, shake the rollette, remove the lid, and roll or dab a little of the liquid across your chosen pulse point (see opposite).

ROLLETTE BLENDS

The combinations below are especially good for rollettes; or you can experiment to find your own favourite blends. All use two drops of each essential oil and 10ml (0.35fl oz) of sunflower oil. Apricot kernel oil can also be used as the base for your blend: both it and sunflower oil are easy to apply as they are lighter and more easily absorbed than most other oils.

For focus and concentration, lime and basil. Use on the temporal pulse point.

To boost energy, lemongrass and rosemary. Use on the apical pulse point.

To revitalize and for motivation, bergamot and bay laurel. Use on the carotid pulse point.

To lift spirits and instill positivity, geranium and sweet orange. Use on the radial pulse point.

BATH AND SHOWER PREPARATIONS

Making your own aromatic bathing products is a simple and natural way to keep your skin nourished and hydrated, and can turn your bath into a spa experience and your morning shower into a vitality-boosting start to the day. There's a range of different ways to use essential oils when bathing, but remember, oil blends will make baths and showers slippy, so be careful when getting in and out.

MINERAL BATH

Adding 2 tbsp of sea salt or Epsom salts and an oil blend to a warm bath will soothe skin and ease stiff joints and aching muscles. Allow the salts to dissolve before you get in.

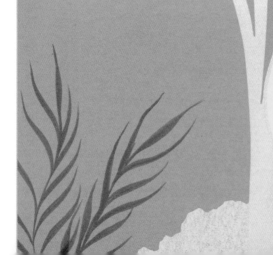

BATH OILS

Blending essential oils with plant oils such as almond or grapeseed is the most common way of enjoying them at bathtime. Add oil blends to an already-run bath to enjoy their aromas and healing properties.

SHOWER GEL

If you use essential oils in a shower gel base, ensure it is natural and unfragranced, and free from sodium lauryl sulphate, a harsh, skin-damaging chemical detergent.

HIP BATH

So-called because you fill a normal bath or container with water to cover your hips, this is a very effective remedy for treating issues such as constipation, cystitis, and haemorrhoids, or to speed post-childbirth healing.

OAT BATH

Placing a small, essential oil-infused parcel of oats in a bath will help improve your skin by softening it, removing dead cells, and drawing out impurities.

BATH MELTS

These usually contain natural butters, which are deeply nourishing to the skin. See pages 72–73 for an indulgent bath-melts recipe.

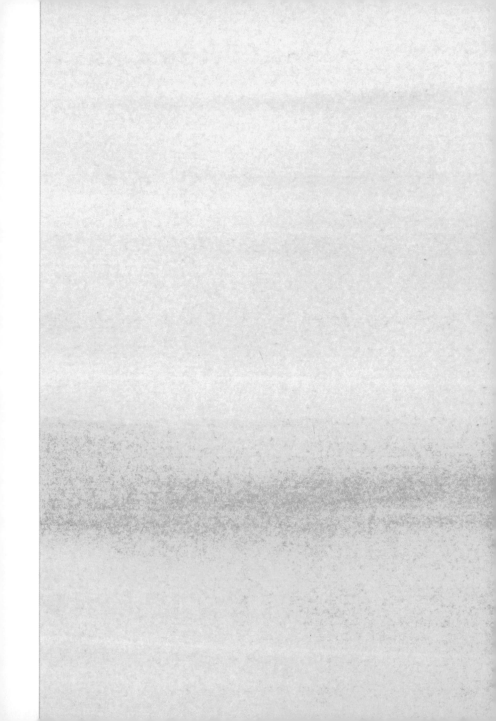

AIR APPLICATIONS

There are several ways in which we can encourage essential oils to release their therapeutic compounds into the air. It's by inhaling these airborne aromas that we take in those compounds, allowing both brain and lungs to be infused with their powerful, transformative properties.

TISSUE

Inhaling a tissue infused with 1–4 drops of calming or energizing essential oil is the easiest way to practise aromatherapy. If you take the tissue with you in a sealable plastic bag, you can inhale it throughout the day. At night, place an oil-infused tissue by your pillow to help you sleep.

AROMASTICK

These lipstick-sized tubes are a handy means of inhaling when you are on the move. To use, unscrew the base of the aromastick and add 10 drops of your chosen essential oil to the cotton wadding inside. Screw the base back on and it's ready to use.

INHALING ESSENTIAL OILS

How can inhaling essential oils make us not just feel better emotionally or mentally, but physically, too? The answer lies in the natural chemicals those aromas contain, how they enter the body, and what happens when they get there.

STEAM INHALATION

This is a traditional home remedy for conditions including congestion and sinusitis. Add 2–4 drops of an essential oil such as eucalyptus globulus to a bowl of hot water, cover your head with a towel, and breathe in the anti-inflammatory, mucus-clearing aromas.

"AMBIENT" INHALATION

However you use essential oils you will also be inhaling their scent, stimulating the limbic area of the brain to produce an emotional or physical response. This amplifies and deepens the holistic effects of your essential oil-enhanced massage, shower, bath, or skin treatment.

AROMATIC "FAMILIES"

Essential oils that share aromatic characteristics are often grouped together. Here are three of the main families:

FRESH includes peppermint, rosemary, tea tree, eucalyptus, lemon, lime.

FLOWERY includes rose, geranium, jasmine, ylang ylang, neroli, lavender.

EARTHY includes sandalwood, myrrh, vetiver, cypress, frankincense.

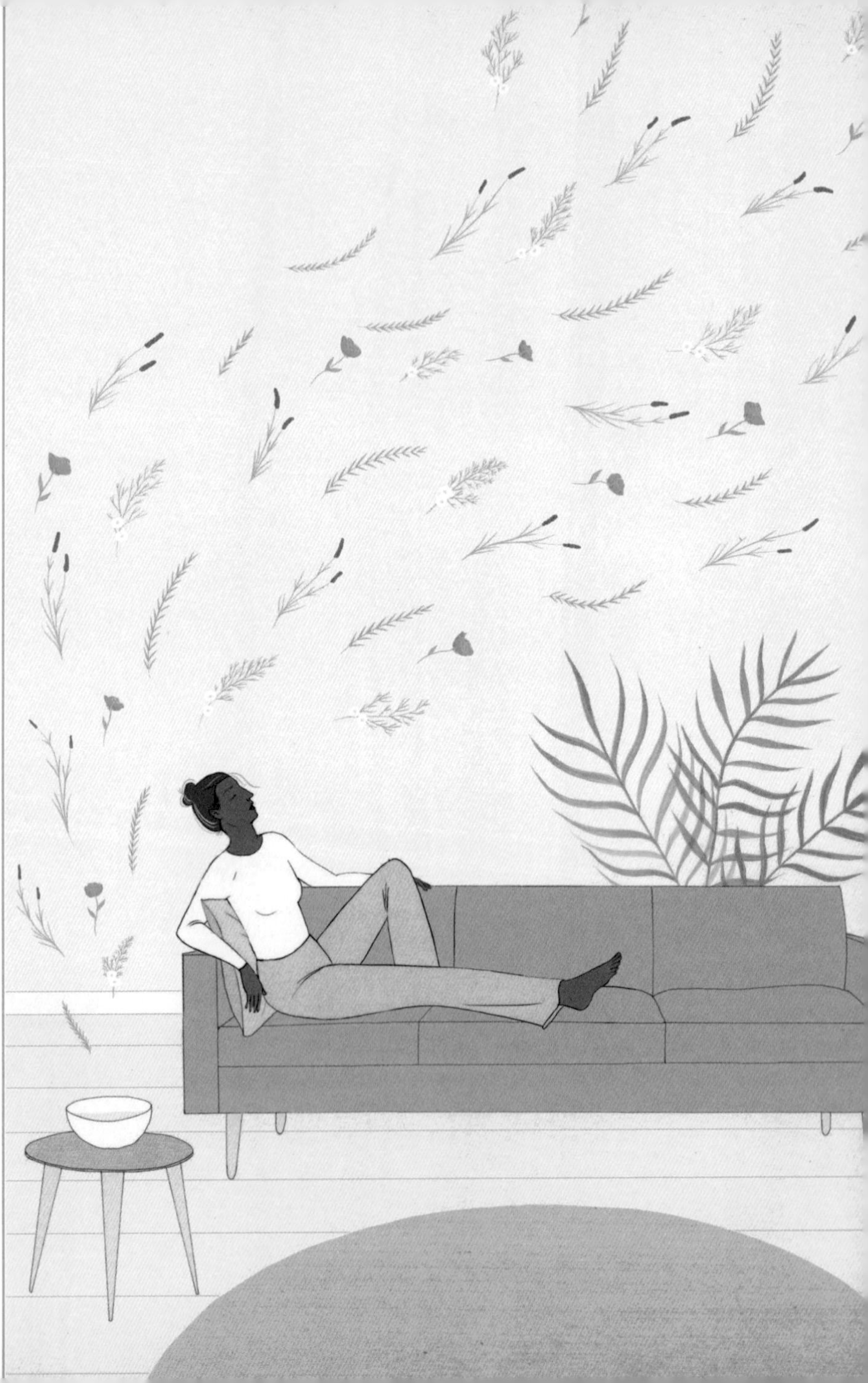

EVAPORATION AND ROOM SPRAYS

Aromatherapy's rewards are often personal, whether it's a healing self-massage or an energizing aromastick. By using sprays or evaporation, you can transform the atmosphere in a room for everybody's benefit.

BOWL EVAPORATION

Evaporation is one of the simplest ways to enjoy aromatherapy, a slow way to release essential oil aromas into the air by adding, for example, two drops each of eucalyptus radiata, lavender, and lemon to a bowl of water and leaving it to infuse. The oils' aromas will slowly develop and linger for at least a couple of days. Place the bowl out of reach of children or pets.

Bowl evaporation works for any environment, but is especially useful where there are lingering odours, or for cleansing a "sick" room where someone has recently been ill and the atmosphere needs to be refreshed.

ROOM SPRAY

Room sprays freshen up rooms fast, get rid of smells, repel insects, or create a relaxing atmosphere before guests arrive. Shake well before each use, and avoid spraying on furniture.

Makes 30ml (1fl oz)

Essential oils:

- 20 drops of your chosen oil blend

Other items:

30ml (1fl oz) of filtered water; spray bottle

How to make

Put the water in the bottle, then add the essential oils. Screw on the lid and shake to combine. Store in a cool, dark place and use within 6 weeks.

USING ROOM DIFFUSERS

Diffusers are an excellent way of scenting a room. There are no complicated practices to master or complex techniques to learn: just put your oils in, fire them up or switch them on, and go.

Diffusers work by dispersing molecules of essential oils into the air. They are easy to use and low-maintenance.

TYPES OF ROOM DIFFUSER

Ultrasonic diffusers create intense vibrations within a mix of water and essential oils, releasing a fine mist into the air. They are mains or battery operated and are quiet and easy to use.

Electronic nebulizers force water into a pressurized atomizer, creating a mist of ultrafine particles that hang in the air for hours, rather than quickly settling, as with other diffusers. They tend to cost more than other diffusers, but are regarded as the most effective. It's this type of diffuser that's used in the examples in this book.

Fan diffusers blow air across an essential oil-infused wick or pad, releasing aromatic particles. They are inexpensive, and are battery or mains operated.

Oil burners work by warming essential oils, causing them to evaporate and diffuse into the air. Traditional burners use small or tea-light candles to warm the

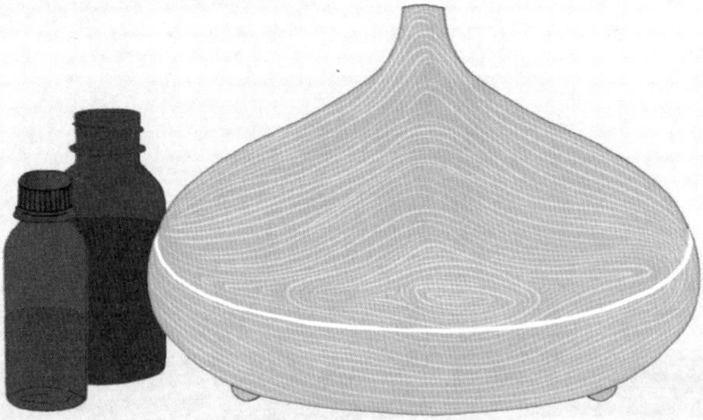

oil, while modern burners contain an electric heat element.
Reed diffusers are sticks part-immersed in oil-infused water. Liquid rises through them by capillary action, dispersing scent into the air.

WHAT ARE THEY GOOD FOR?

Relaxation and sleep Rose and lavender are excellent for promoting rest.
Respiratory health Use anti-inflammatory oils such as tea tree and eucalyptus.
Room fresheners Grapefruit or bergamot dissipate musty, stale, or smoky smells.
Enhancing mood Lemon stimulates the brain to produce happy-making serotonin.
Reducing stress and anxiety Try calming neroli and bergamot.
Bug repellent Peppermint and cedarwood are both good options.
Increasing energy Rosemary and orange are especially energizing oils.
Strengthening immunity Litsea and thyme are antibacterial and antiviral.
Boosting memory and focus Basil and rosemary help combat forgetfulness.

TREATMENTS AND BLENDS

WELLBEING TREATMENTS

In the pages that follow you'll discover simple ways you can use essential oils to transform the way you feel; lifting your mood when you feel low, clearing a clouded brain, restoring emotional and mental balance, relieving anxiety and stress, and rejuvenating a tired body and mind.

MORNING MEDITATION

Starting your day with meditation – focusing the mind in order to achieve calm and clarity – banishes the fog of sleep and sets you up for the day ahead. In this simple breathing meditation, inhaling the sweet, bracing scent of limes will help you to keep your attention on your breath throughout the practice.

01

Put a couple of drops of lime essential oil on a tissue. Lime has a good balance of calming and uplifting properties.

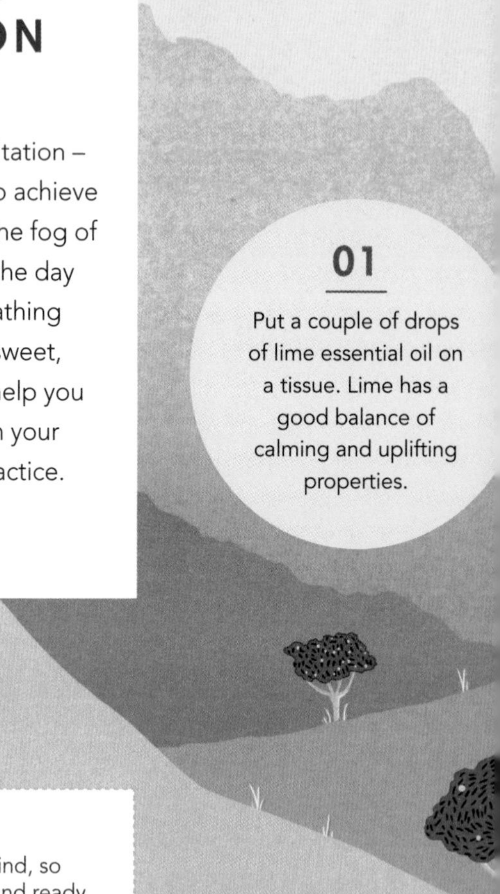

NEED TO KNOW

BENEFITS Clears and calms the mind, so that you begin the day grounded and ready for whatever lies ahead.

TIME 5–10 minutes daily, after waking.

PREPARATION In a quiet place, sit comfortably on a chair, or on the floor.

ITEMS NEEDED 2 drops of lime essential oil; a tissue; a mat or a blanket to sit on, or a chair.

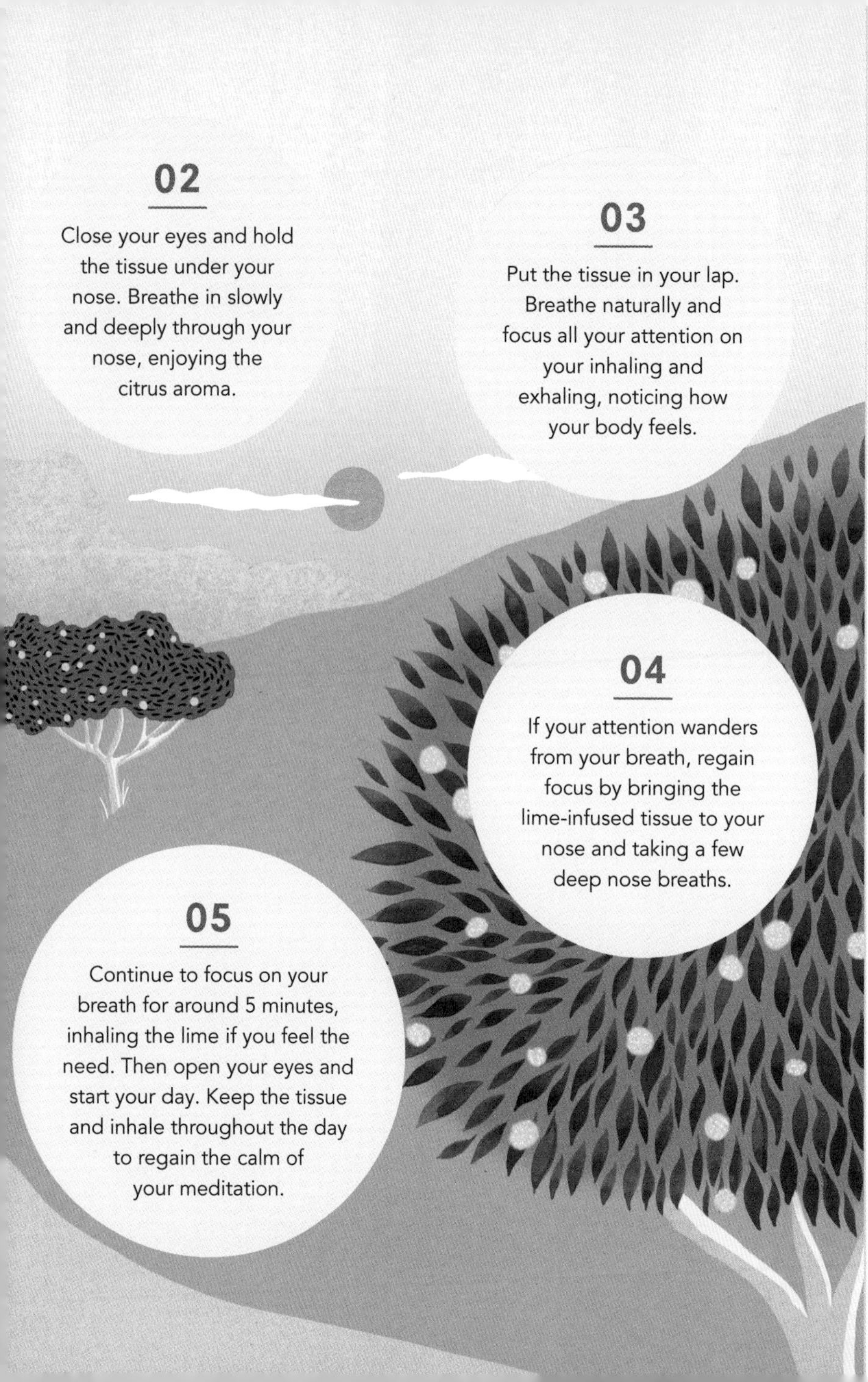

02

Close your eyes and hold the tissue under your nose. Breathe in slowly and deeply through your nose, enjoying the citrus aroma.

03

Put the tissue in your lap. Breathe naturally and focus all your attention on your inhaling and exhaling, noticing how your body feels.

04

If your attention wanders from your breath, regain focus by bringing the lime-infused tissue to your nose and taking a few deep nose breaths.

05

Continue to focus on your breath for around 5 minutes, inhaling the lime if you feel the need. Then open your eyes and start your day. Keep the tissue and inhale throughout the day to regain the calm of your meditation.

01

Avoiding broken or delicate skin, begin by brushing the soles of your feet, then work up to your thighs and buttocks, using long upward strokes. Repeat 3 times on each leg.

02

Make long sweeping strokes across the buttocks and towards the middle of the back. Repeat 3 times on each side. Then, gently brush the stomach in a clockwise direction.

DETOX BRUSH AND SHOWER ROUTINE

Dry skin brushing is a great way to eliminate toxins, boost circulation, and naturally exfoliate. Follow up with a supercharged shower blend of detoxing and cleansing essential oils and you will feel radiant all day.

03

Brush your arms, from wrists to shoulders. Finally, brush across your shoulders and down your back.

04

Now take a warm shower. Pour a little of the shower blend onto a sponge or flannel, and breathe in its invigorating aroma.

05

Massage the blend into your skin and rinse off. Finish by taking a few last breaths of the warm, scented air.

NEED TO KNOW

BENEFITS Stimulates circulation and lymphatic systems, boosting energy and vitality.

TIME 5 minutes each for brushing and shower.

ITEMS NEEDED Long-handled body brush; "Wake-up shower gel" blend (see pages 68–69; you could also substitute its essential oils for geranium, juniper, and lemon – or create your own blend).

RESTORE BALANCE

We all occasionally lose our equilibrium, which can leave us mentally or physically drained. These essential oil blends will restore your mind-body balance and help you feel grounded again.

Our bodies and minds naturally seek balance. When we feel out of sorts, sometimes we simply need to pause and make space for the body to do its job and restore harmony. Essential oils can help with this process and the selections used in these three blends have uplifting, thought-clarifying, restorative, and relaxing qualities that will brighten your mood and leave you feeling healthier and more composed.

BEST BALANCING ESSENTIAL OILS

Lavender	Sweet orange
Cypress	Mandarin
Rose	Sandalwood
Palmarosa	Cedarwood atlas
Geranium	Frankincense

RESTORATIVE ROOM DIFFUSION

Use this emotionally balancing room blend in the early evening to help you reset at the end of a long day.

Makes 1 diffusion

Essential oils:

- 2 drops of cypress
- 2 drops of geranium
- 2 drops of sweet orange

Other items:

Room diffuser

How to make

Add the recommended amount of water to the diffuser, then add the drops of essential oils to the surface of the water.

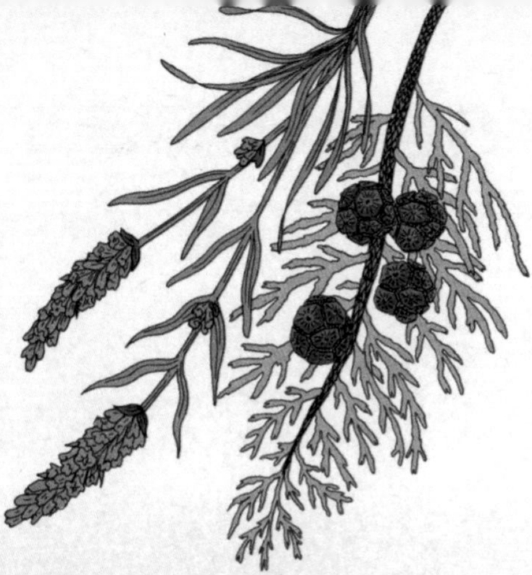

AROMATIC BATH SOAK

Lavender is a restorative, while palmarosa refreshes and cedarwood strengthens. Blending them with almond oil helps to moisturize dry skin.

Makes 1 bath blend

Essential oils:

- 3 drops of cedarwood atlas
- 3 drops of palmarosa
- 4 drops of lavender

Other items:

20ml (0.7fl oz) of almond oil or unfragranced bath foamer base

How to make

Mix the essential oils with your chosen base and add to a warm bath.

NIGHT MASSAGE OIL

Before bed, massage your body with this soothing blend of thought-settling mandarin and relaxing frankincense and sandalwood.

Makes 30ml (1fl oz)

Essential oils:

- 3 drops of sandalwood
- 6 drops of frankincense
- 6 drops of mandarin

Other items:

30ml (1fl oz) of grapeseed oil; small bottle with lid

How to make

Pour the grapeseed oil into the bottle then add the essential oils. Put the lid on and combine. This is a body blend, so avoid using on the face (see pages 22–23).

01

To make the oat bag, put the oats either in the centre of the muslin, or in the "tights" bag. Add the essential oils and tie into a tight parcel.

02

Run a warm bath, letting the oat parcel float in the water as the bath fills.

03

Soak in the bath for 20 minutes, inhaling the calming aromas and enjoying the sensation of your skin feeling soothed and nourished.

SKIN-SOOTHING OAT BATH

Combine antibacterial lavender, soothing Roman chamomile, and nourishing oats in a bath soak to calm itchy, dry skin. Oats contain saponins (gentle natural cleansers), and their pH (acidity level) balances the inflammatory, drying effects of high-pH, alkaline water.

05

Lie back and relax for a few more minutes, taking time to fully appreciate the sense of wellbeing that your blissful bath time-out has created.

04

If you wish, take the oat parcel and gently rub it all over your body to exfoliate the skin and stimulate circulation.

NEED TO KNOW

BENEFITS Oats soothe and rebalance skin. The essential oil will leave you feeling cool, calm, and content.

TIME 30 minutes.

ITEMS NEEDED Essential oils: 2 drops each of lavender and Roman chamomile; 4 tbsp rolled oats; 15cm (6in) muslin square, or the cut-off foot of an old pair of tights; string to secure the bag.

IMMUNITY-BOOSTING MASSAGE

Studies show that massage can increase the number of disease-fighting white blood cells in the body, while certain essential oils are also proven to support the immune system. This chest massage will strengthen your body's ability to fight off illness.

NEED TO KNOW

BENEFITS Stimulates the production of lymphocytes (immune cells) in the thymus at the base of the throat, one of your immune system's primary glands. Also releases both mental and upper-body muscular tension.

TIME 5 minutes; perform twice daily.

PREPARATION Blend 30ml (1fl oz) of grapeseed oil in a small bottle with 3 drops of thyme and 5 drops each of litsea and niaouli essential oils.

01

Warm 3–4 drops of the massage oil in your palms. Cup your hands over your face and inhale slowly, enjoying the fresh, uplifting aroma.

02

Using your fingertips, begin at the base of your throat and massage out towards your shoulder, then around your chest, and back to the base of your throat. Do this for 2–3 minutes, pressing firmly but without causing discomfort.

03

Warm a few more drops of oil in your hands and, using your palms, lightly rub your neck and shoulders for a minute or two. Finally, enjoy inhaling the fresh, citrussy aromas as the oil absorbs into your skin.

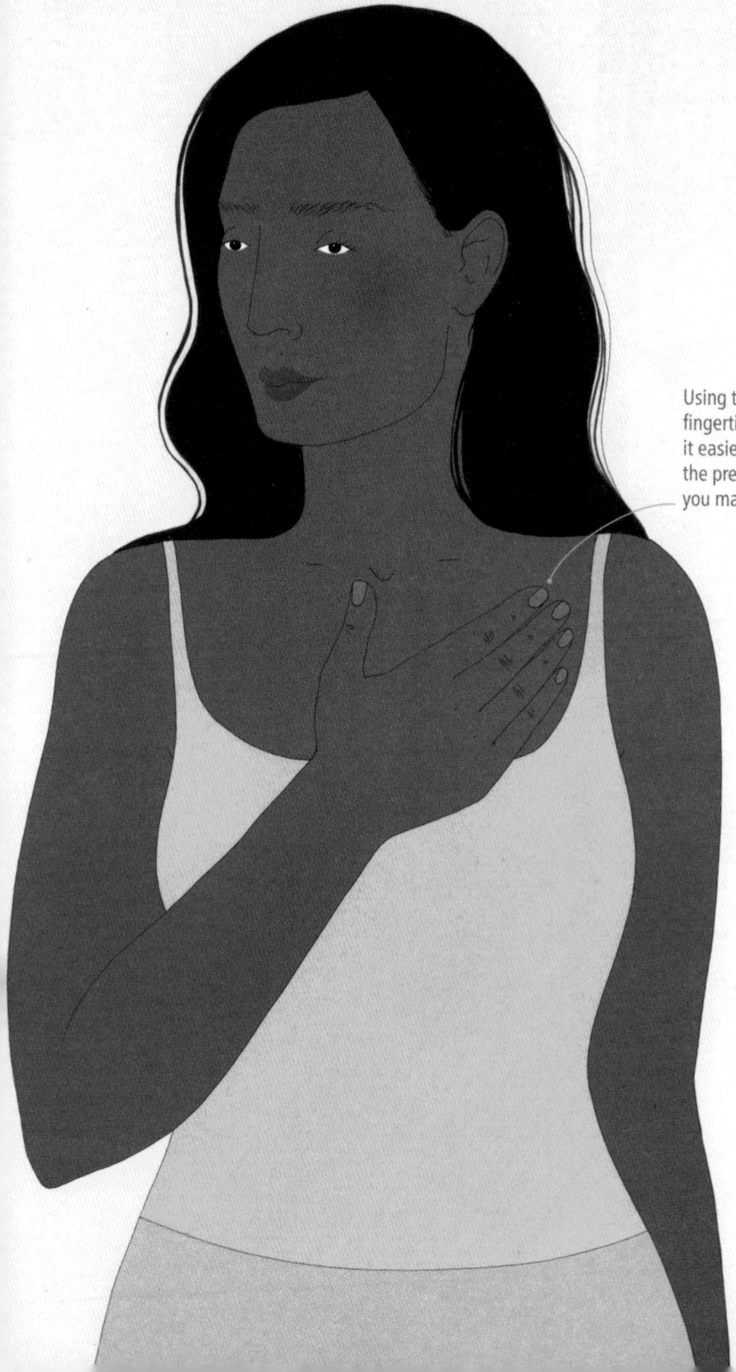

Using the fingertips makes it easier to control the pressure as you massage

ENERGIZING BLENDS

When you need a quick burst of energy, there are powerful essential oils that will give you the boost you need until you can properly rest and restore yourself.

Mental and physical exhaustion is often the result of a busy or demanding lifestyle. Other factors such as insomnia, stress, trauma, or poor eating habits, and too much or too little exercise, can also drain your resources. The blends here are a natural, healthy equivalent of a caffeine hit, combining herbal and refreshing essential oils in combinations that will revive and deliver a quick, sustainable boost to your system.

BEST ENERGIZING ESSENTIAL OILS

Sweet basil	Lemon
Black pepper	Grapefruit
Black spruce	Geranium
Rosemary	Lemongrass
Ginger	Thyme

ENERGY-BURST AROMASTICK

Inhaling this blend delivers an immediate pick-me-up, as all these essential oils have refreshing, uplifting properties.

Makes 1 aromastick

Essential oils:

- 2 drops of basil
- 2 drops of ravensara
- 2 drops of thyme
- 4 drops of lime

Other items:

Aromastick

How to make

Add essential oils to the aromastick. Inhale throughout the day as required.

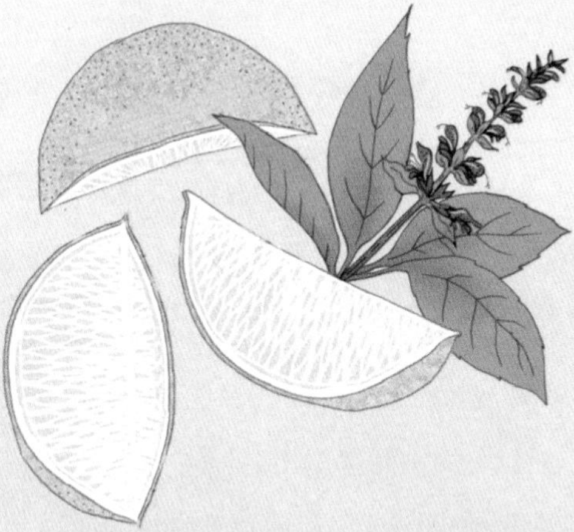

ROLL-ON FATIGUE BUSTER

Dab this on your wrists and other pulse points whenever fatigue strikes. Calming geranium balances refreshing grapefruit and gently revitalizing clary sage.

Makes 10ml (0.35fl oz)

Essential oils:

- 2 drops of clary sage
- 3 drops of grapefruit
- 4 drops of geranium

Other items:

Rollette bottle; 10ml (0.35fl oz) of sunflower oil

How to make

Pour the sunflower oil into the bottle then add the essential oils. Put the lid on and shake to combine (see pages 38–39 for more on using rollette bottles).

REVITALIZING EAR MASSAGE

Ear massage is used in traditional Chinese medicine to stimulate energy (*chi*) to flow through the body's channels. Add a few drops of this blend to your thumb and index fingertips then gently rub the ear, starting at the top and working down to the earlobe. Repeat for the other ear.

Makes 30ml (1fl oz)

Essential oils:

- 3 drops of black spruce
- 3 drops of geranium

Other items:

30ml (1fl oz) of grapeseed oil; small plastic bottle with lid

How to make

Pour the oil into the bottle then add the essential oils. Put the lid on and shake to combine.

BREATHING FOR SELF-CONFIDENCE

Lack of confidence shows in how we carry ourselves – when we slump, our breath gets shallower and we feel even worse. This breathing exercise, accompanied by energizing grapefruit oil, will help you regain your sparkle and stand tall again.

NEED TO KNOW

BENEFITS Encourages a more upright, outward-looking posture; boosts the body's oxygen intake; lifts mood.

TIME 5 minutes daily, or whenever confidence is low.

PREPARATION In a quiet place, stand with your feet a hips' width apart.

ITEMS NEEDED
2 drops of grapefruit essential oil; a tissue.

01

Put the oil onto the tissue and hold it under your nose. Close your eyes and slowly breathe in and out, savouring the fresh, uplifting aroma.

02

Put your hand on your stomach. Breathe in and out, deep into your abdomen, feeling it rise and fall. Now move your hand to your chest and again breathe deeply, feeling your hand rise and fall with each breath.

03

Alternate the abdomen and chest breathing for about 5 minutes, until you feel your body is expanded and open. Keep the tissue and inhale it throughout the day to revisit that liberating sensation.

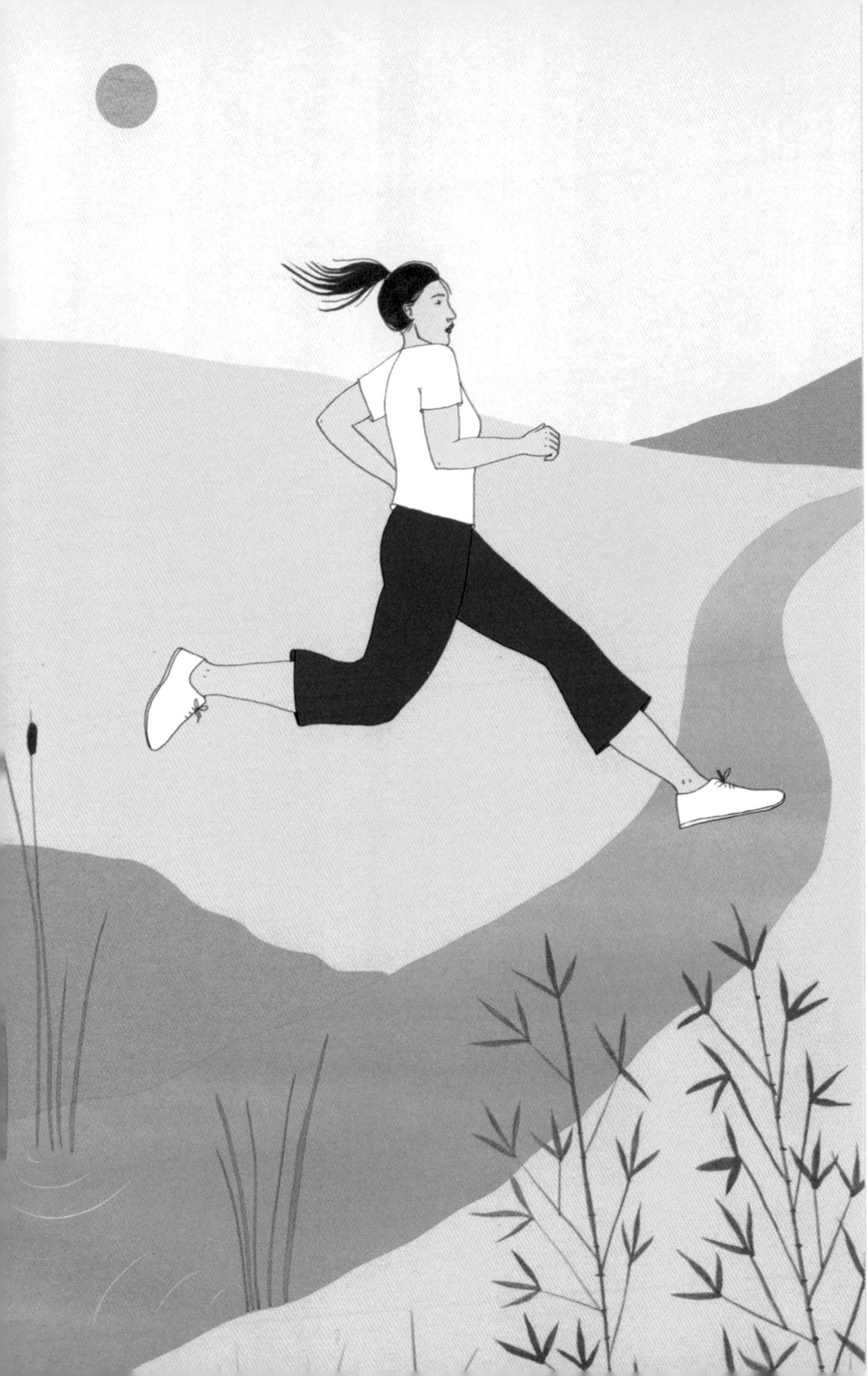

BOOST FOCUS AND CONCENTRATION

Studies show that essential oils can have a marked effect on our thinking processes and memory. Use these blends whenever you need to sharpen your focus.

So much to do, so little time! It's easy to lose your edge when chores mount up or you're in the middle of a demanding task. These blends have been specially selected for their abilities to restore alertness, clear your headspace, or focus a wandering mind. All three feature rosemary essential oil, which has a stimulating effect on the central nervous system and really helps with concentration in particular.

BEST ESSENTIAL OILS FOR FOCUS

Rosemary	Grapefruit
Basil	Sweet orange
Peppermint	Geranium
Thyme	Black pepper
Lemon	Bergamot

WAKE-UP SHOWER GEL

Awaken your senses and sharpen your mind for the day ahead with this powerful, zesty, and citrussy blend.

Makes 100ml (3.5fl oz)

Essential oils:

- 10 drops of black pepper
- 10 drops of grapefruit
- 10 drops of rosemary
- 10 drops of sweet orange

Other items:

100ml (3.5fl oz) of unfragranced shower gel; small bottle with lid

How to make

Add the essential oils and the shower gel to the bottle and shake to combine. Use as necessary.

BRAIN-TONIC ROLLER BLEND

Use this on your pulse points through the day. The black pepper combats mental fatigue, and is especially useful if you're studying.

Makes 10ml (0.35fl oz)

Essential oils:

- 2 drops of black pepper
- 2 drops of geranium
- 2 drops of rosemary

Other items:

10ml (0.35fl oz) glass rollette bottle; 10ml (0.35fl oz) of sunflower oil

How to make

Pour the sunflower oil into the bottle and add the essential oils. Screw the lid on and shake to combine.

FOCUS FAST AROMASTICK

This blend of instantly reviving and invigorating oils will clear your mind when your brain begins to fog.

Makes 1 aromastick

Essential oils:

- 2 drops of peppermint
- 3 drops of lemon
- 3 drops of rosemary

Other items:

Aromastick

How to make

Add the essential oils to the aromastick. Inhale whenever you feel your concentration start to waver.

SENSUAL BLENDS

Get that loving feeling back on track with these warm, indulgent, and luxurious blends that will help you explore and enjoy your sensuality.

Use the blends here to bring you comfort and calm, allowing you to create the space to feel love and joy, and to release your natural sexual energy. Rose and jasmine essential oils are sweet, floral, and beautifully intoxicating. Sandalwood is emotionally grounding, and floral ylang ylang is uniquely uplifting and arousing.

BEST SENSUAL ESSENTIAL OILS

Rose	Cardamom
Jasmine	Geranium
Clary sage	Frankincense
Ylang ylang	Sandalwood
Patchouli	Cedarwood

STIMULATING ROOM SCENT

Create an arousing atmosphere with this subtle, sensual room blend. Turn on the diffuser 30 minutes before you go to bed to ensure its scents completely fill your bedroom.

Makes 1 diffusion

Essential oils:

- 1 drop of ylang ylang
- 2 drops of black pepper
- 3 drops of mandarin

Other items:

Room diffuser

How to make

Add the recommended amount of water to the diffuser, then add the drops of essential oils to the surface of the water.

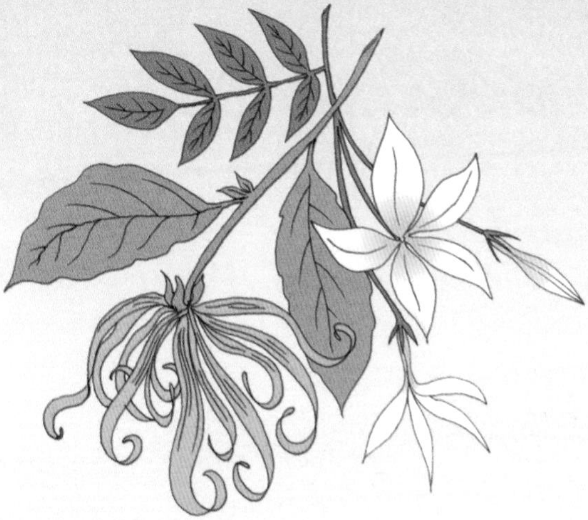

ROMANTIC BATH SOAK

Especially effective for women, this profoundly floral blend can help turn your thoughts to sensual pleasure as you luxuriate in the silky, fragrant water.

Makes 1 bath blend

Essential oils:

- 3 drops of geranium
- 3 drops of rose
- 4 drops of frankincense

Other items:

20ml (0.7fl oz) of almond oil, milk, or unfragranced bath foamer base

How to make

Mix the essential oils with your chosen base and add to a warm bath.

LOVING TOUCH MASSAGE OIL

You and your partner can use this heady blend to massage each other as part of your lovemaking.

Makes 1 massage blend

Essential oils:

- 2 drops of jasmine
- 3 drops of cardamom
- 3 drops of sandalwood

Other items:

30ml (1fl oz) of grapeseed oil; small bottle with lid

How to make

Pour the oil into the bottle then add the essential oils. Put the lid on and shake to combine.

BATH MELTS FOR PREGNANCY

These luxurious bath melts contain essential oils to calm your body and mind as well as shea butter and moisturizing coconut oil to nourish your skin during pregnancy. To use, add a melt to warm, running bath water, or gently rub one on your skin when taking a warm shower.

01

Place a bowl over a pan of gently simmering water. Add the shea and cocoa butters to the bowl and let them melt together. Take care to not let the water boil.

NEED TO KNOW

BENEFITS Geranium and lavender balance pregnancy hormones and help keep skin supple.

TIME 5 minutes to make; at least 1 hour to cool and set.

ITEMS NEEDED *Makes 10 melts:* 25g (0.8fl oz) each of shea and cocoa butters; 1 tbsp of coconut oil; 5 drops each of geranium and lavender essential oils; saucepan; heatproof bowl; silicon tray of mini cupcake moulds or individual paper cases; cotton bag; geranium flowers (optional).

CAUTION Melts can make baths or showers slippy, so take care. If you are pregnant, make sure the water is warm, not hot.

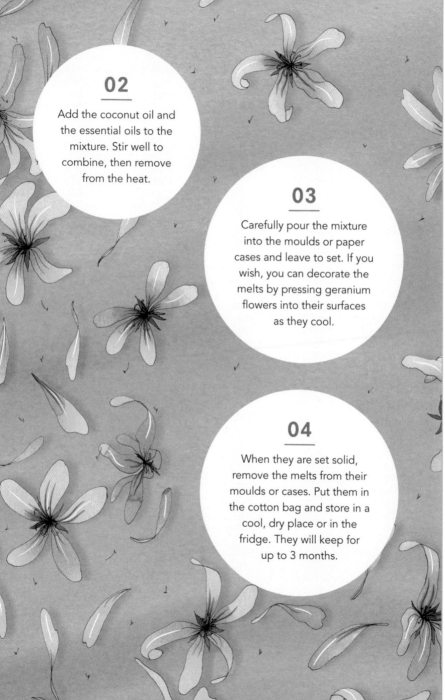

02

Add the coconut oil and the essential oils to the mixture. Stir well to combine, then remove from the heat.

03

Carefully pour the mixture into the moulds or paper cases and leave to set. If you wish, you can decorate the melts by pressing geranium flowers into their surfaces as they cool.

04

When they are set solid, remove the melts from their moulds or cases. Put them in the cotton bag and store in a cool, dry place or in the fridge. They will keep for up to 3 months.

BEST UPLIFTING ESSENTIAL OILS

- Rosemary
- Mandarin
- Ylang ylang
- Thyme
- Bergamot
- Black pepper
- Neroli
- Rose
- Basil
- Lemon

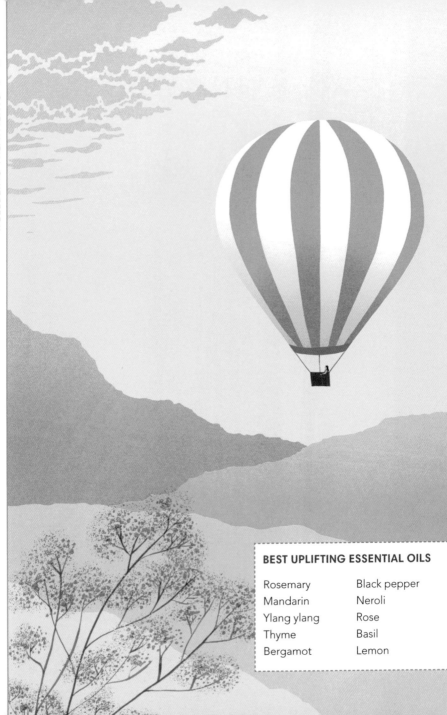

LIFT YOUR MOOD

Everything within and around us is made of molecules that vibrate at different frequencies – and the higher the frequency the happier we feel. Research shows that essential oils have the highest frequencies in nature, so breathe in these joyful blends, feel connected – and smile!

GOOD VIBRATIONS SHOWER GEL

Raise your spirits with this herby and mildly citrussy shower blend. Use it on the body only, avoiding the face.

Makes 100ml (3.5fl oz)

Essential oils:

- 10 drops of ylang ylang
- 20 drops of bergamot
- 20 drops of rosemary
- 20 drops of thyme

Other items:

100ml (3.5fl oz) of unfragranced shower gel; small bottle with lid

How to make

Add the essential oils and gel to the bottle and shake to combine. Use as necessary.

UPLIFTING AROMASTICK

This intense blend of herbal, zesty, and spicy aromas will add sunshine to your day.

Makes 1 aromastick

Essential oils:

- 2 drops of basil
- 3 drops of patchouli
- 5 drops of lemon

Other items:

Aromastick

How to make

Add the essential oils to the aromastick. Inhale throughout the day as required.

01

Sitting up comfortably, rest the sole of your left foot on your right knee. Using both hands, massage a little oil all over your left foot.

02

Using your thumbs, massage the sole of the foot with circular motions. If an area feels sensitive or tight, go over it a few times to release and relax the muscles.

03

With an open palm, make long, firm strokes along the sole from heel to toe. This improves circulation and calms anxiety.

REFLEXOLOGY FOOT MASSAGE

This exercise is based on the practice of reflexology, in which massaging energy channels in the feet has beneficial balancing effects on the body. This massage will refresh the feet, help you to relax, and ward off fungal infections, too.

05

Repeat steps 1–4 on your other foot. Finally, cover your feet with cotton socks, allowing the oil to penetrate and soften the skin overnight.

04

Slowly rub the top of the foot with your thumbs. Gently squeeze and rotate each toe, especially the big toe, which is linked in reflexology to the sleep-promoting pineal gland. Then massage around the ankle bone. End with sweeping strokes from your ankle to your toes.

NEED TO KNOW

BENEFITS Stimulates pineal gland to promote better sleep; improves digestion and blood flow.

TIME About 10 minutes.

PREPARATION Add 2 drops of tea tree oil to a bowl of warm water; soak your feet for 5 minutes.

ITEMS NEEDED Use the "Calming massage oil" blend on pages 124–125.

MANAGE GRIEF

When you're grieving, emotions such as anxiety, guilt, overwhelming sadness, and even anger can hit – often when you least expect them. These soothing blends can help you feel more grounded and stable during bleak times.

RESCUE REMEDY AROMASTICK

When grief threatens to overwhelm you, this blend, containing beautiful, floral neroli, will instantly calm and soothe your spirits.

Makes 1 aromastick

Essential oils:

- 3 drops of bergamot
- 3 drops of mandarin
- 4 drops of neroli

Other items:

Aromastick

How to make

Add the essential oils to the aromastick. Inhale throughout the day as required.

RESTORING BATH SOAK

This blend contains frankincense and cypress, often called transition oils for their effectiveness during times of change or upheaval.

Makes 1 bath blend

Essential oils:

- 3 drops of cypress
- 3 drops of rose
- 4 drops of frankincense

Other items:

20ml (0.7fl oz) of almond oil, milk, or unfragranced bath foamer base

How to make

Mix the essential oils with your chosen base and add to a warm bath.

BEST ESSENTIAL OILS FOR GRIEF

Neroli
Cypress
Frankincense
Bergamot
Mandarin
Yarrow
Myrrh
Rose
Myrtle
Clary sage

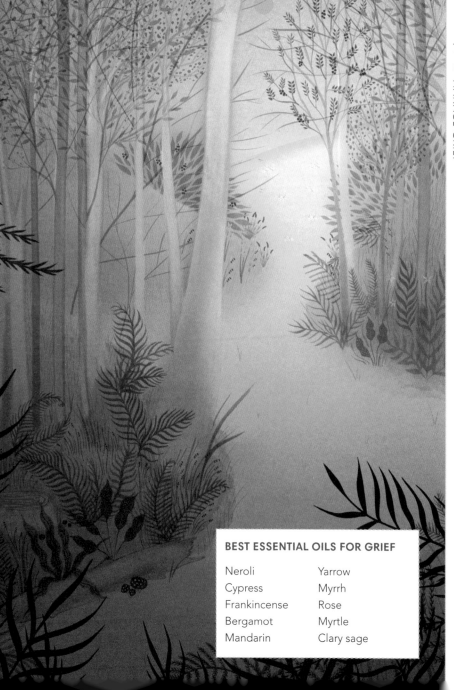

BEST STRESS-BUSTING ESSENTIAL OILS

- Black spruce
- Sweet basil
- Neroli
- Patchouli
- Lavender
- Roman chamomile
- Bergamot
- Cedarwood atlas
- Frankincense
- Rose

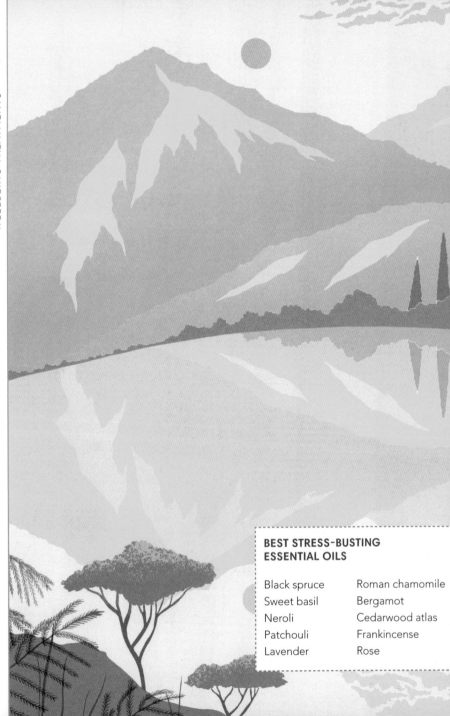

TURN DOWN THE STRESS DIAL

While some stress can be helpful and motivating, too much for too long can affect your sleep, digestion, and ability to enjoy life. When stress levels soar, these blends will calm your thoughts and slow your breath, helping you to regain your natural balance.

INSTANT STRESS-BUSTER

Inhale this through the day whenever stress levels rise. Sweet basil will bring you back to the present, bergamot is uplifting and frankincense revitalizes.

Makes 1 aromastick

Essential oils:

- 2 drops of basil
- 3 drops of bergamot
- 3 drops of frankincense

Other items:

Aromastick

How to make

Add the essential oils to the aromastick. Inhale throughout the day as required.

UNWINDING BATH SOAK

These comforting oils are perfect for an evening bath blend, cocooning you in feelings of calm and relaxation.

Makes 1 bath blend

Essential oils:

- 3 drops of Roman chamomile
- 3 drops of rose
- 4 drops of lavender

Other items:

20ml (0.7fl oz) of almond oil, milk, or unfragranced bath foamer base

How to make

Mix the essential oils with your chosen base and add to a warm bath.

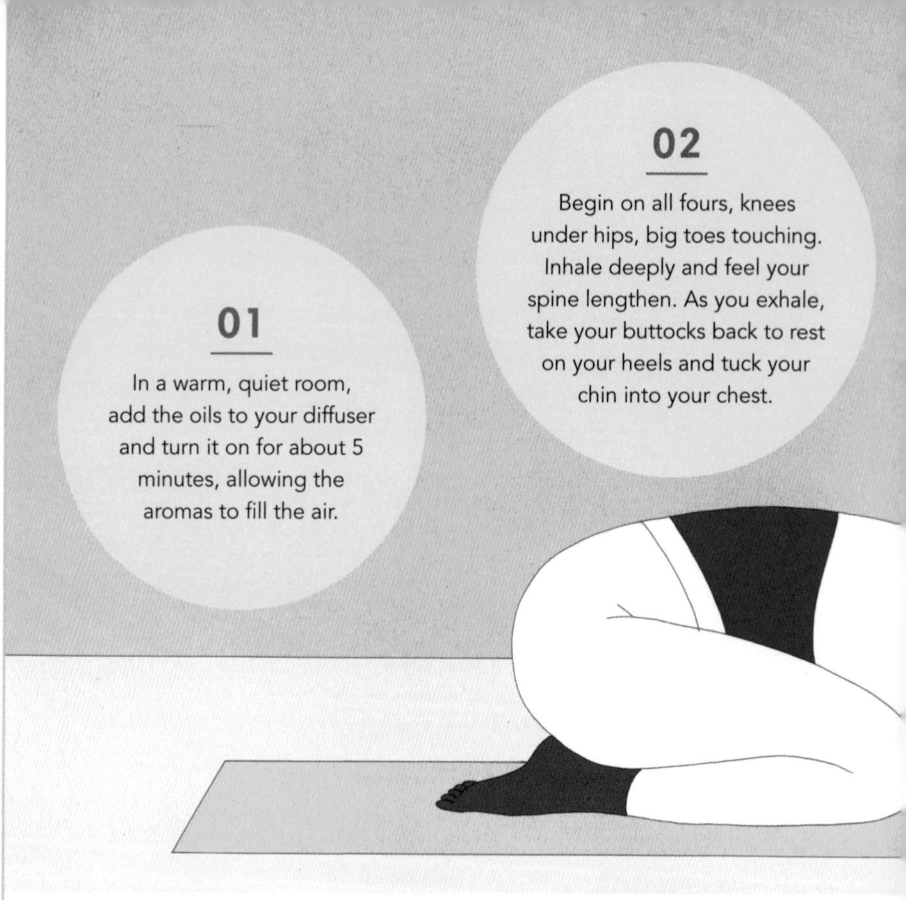

01

In a warm, quiet room, add the oils to your diffuser and turn it on for about 5 minutes, allowing the aromas to fill the air.

02

Begin on all fours, knees under hips, big toes touching. Inhale deeply and feel your spine lengthen. As you exhale, take your buttocks back to rest on your heels and tuck your chin into your chest.

RESTORATIVE YOGA STRETCH

Balasana, or child's pose, is a yoga position that calms the brain and relieves fatigue. Infusing the room with essential oil aromas enhances your practice, whether it's an energizing morning stretch or an evening wind-down.

03

Rest with your forehead on the ground and arms outstretched. If it's more comfortable, put your arms next to your body, palms up.

04

Breathe deeply, taking in the aromas of your chosen oil. Stay in this position for about 5 minutes, or as long as you feel comfortable.

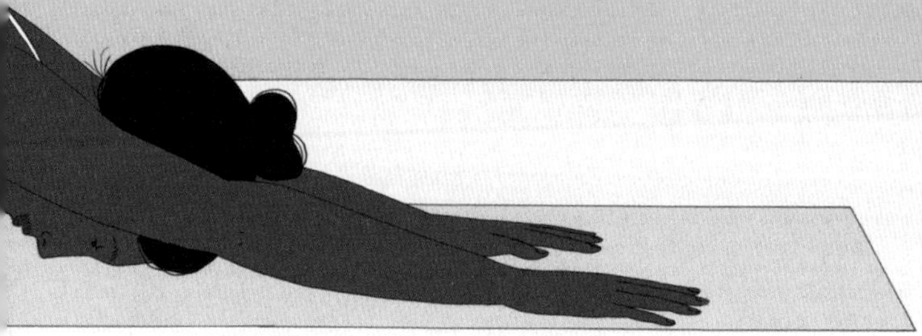

NEED TO KNOW

BENEFITS Gently stretches hip and pelvic area; relieves mental stress; eases joint pain.

TIME About 5–10 minutes, morning or night.

EQUIPMENT NEEDED Yoga mat or a rug to protect your knees; diffuser (see pages 48–49).
Morning stretch: 2 drops each of geranium and sweet orange.
Evening stretch: 2 drops each of lavender and patchouli.

FRAGRANT FACIAL OILS

Facial oils are simple to make, and the essential oils help to balance the oil levels of all skin types, whether dry, combination, spotty, or oily.

You can combine essential oils with plant oils to make effective facial massage blends. Plant oils such as evening primrose, argan, and avocado contain fatty acids, vitamins, and minerals which have replenishing and regenerative properties. See pages 90–91 for instructions on how to perform a facial massage that you can use for all three of these blends.

BEST FACIAL ESSENTIAL OILS

Normal, dry, and/or mature skin:

Rose	Lavender
Neroli	Frankincense

Oily or combination skin:

Palmarosa	Lemon
Lavender	Sandalwood
Geranium	Neroli

NOURISHING BLEND

For normal and dry skin

This enriching mix of essential and plant oils will nourish and balance your skin, giving it a radiant glow. Use morning and night, after cleansing.

Makes 30ml (1fl oz)

Essential oils:

- 2 drops of frankincense
- 2 drops of geranium
- 2 drops of rose

Other items:

5ml (0.2fl oz) of evening primrose oil;
5ml (0.2fl oz) of rosehip oil;
20ml (0.7fl oz) of apricot kernel oil;
small bottle with lid

How to make

Pour the plant oils into the bottle, add the essential oils and combine. Keep the bottle in a cool, dark place when not in use.

BALANCING BLEND

For normal, combination, and oily skin
It may seem contradictory, but essential oils can help balance the skin and reduce oiliness. Use this blend morning and night, on its own or under a moisturizer.

Makes 30ml (1fl oz)

Essential oils:
- 2 drops of geranium
- 2 drops of lavender
- 2 drops of palmarosa

Other items:
5ml (0.2fl oz) of hazelnut oil; 5ml (0.2fl oz) of jojoba oil; 20ml (0.7fl oz) of grapeseed oil; small bottle with lid

How to make

Follow the instructions for the "Nourishing blend" (left).

ANTI-AGING BLEND

For very dry or mature skin
This blend soothes, strengthens, cleanses, and tones the skin. The apricot, argan, and avocado oils will make your skin feel smoother, plumper, and radiant. Use morning and night, on its own or under a moisturizer.

Makes 30ml (1fl oz)

Essential oils:
- 2 drops of frankincense
- 2 drops of myrrh
- 2 drops of rose

Other items:
5ml (0.2fl oz) of argan oil; 5ml (0.2fl oz) of avocado oil; 20ml (0.7fl oz) of apricot kernel oil; small bottle with lid

How to make

Follow the instructions for the "Nourishing blend" (left).

NOURISH HARDWORKING HANDS

Hand creams can deliver a quick aromatherapy shot throughout the day, the essential oils both nourishing and protecting the skin and uplifting and balancing your spirits.

We put our hands through a lot, exposing them to the elements, plunging them in and out of hot and cold water, and subjecting them to soaps and detergents. They deserve the best of care, and enriching a moisturizing base cream with nourishing plant oils and aromatic essential oils does just that, delivering a triple hit of benefits. The three blends here have been specially created to revive and repair your hands at different times of the day.

BEST ESSENTIAL OILS FOR HANDS

Lavender	Myrrh
Rose	Roman chamomile
Patchouli	Ylang ylang
Melissa	Vetiver

UPLIFTING MORNING CREAM

Fragrant ylang ylang and zesty lime will sharpen your senses at the start of the day.

Makes 50g (1.8oz)

Essential oils:

- 5 drops of myrrh
- 8 drops of lime
- 5 drops of ylang ylang

Other items:

5g (0.2oz) of jojoba oil; 45g (1.6oz) of unfragranced cream base; jar with lid

How to make

Place the cream base and jojoba in the jar. Stir to combine, add the essential oils, and stir again.

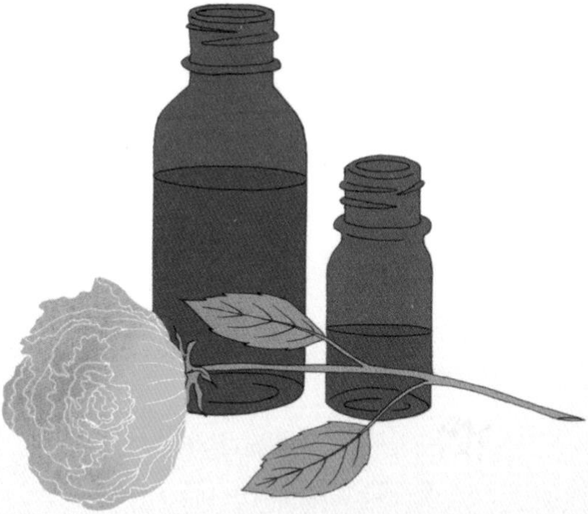

ALL-DAY HAND REPAIR

Overworked, sore hands will love this softening and restorative blend. Use after washing your hands or as necessary.

Makes 50g (1.8oz)

Essential oils:

- 6 drops of patchouli
- 6 drops of Roman chamomile
- 8 drops of lavender

Other items:

5g (0.2oz) of calendula macerated oil; 45g (1.6oz) of unfragranced cream base; jar with lid

How to make

Place the calendula oil and cream base in the jar. Stir to combine, add the essential oils, and stir again.

NOURISHING NIGHT CREAM

This deeply moisturizing cream helps repair and nourish hands overnight. The calming aromas will help you sleep better, too.

Makes 50g (1.8oz)

Essential oils:

- 3 drops of vetiver
- 6 drops of rose
- 8 drops of lavender

Other items:

5g (0.2oz) of rosehip oil; 45g (1.6oz) of unfragranced cream base; jar with lid

How to make

Place the rosehip oil and cream base in the jar. Stir to combine, add the essential oils, and stir again.

01

As you run a warm bath, gently rub the massage oil all over your body, avoiding the face. Tired, aching muscles will start to soothe and flagging spirits begin to revive.

02

When the bath is ready, add the essential oils to it and get in, soaking for at least 20 minutes. The massage oil on your body will merge and intensify with the bath oils, relaxing you further still.

UNWINDING BATH RITUAL

When your busy day is over pamper yourself with this relaxing regime of an aromatherapy self-massage followed by a bath infused with the same soothing essential oils. It's a double hit that will revive and restore you in mind and body.

03

Bring your knees up, feet flat on the bottom of the bath, then lean forward, rounding your back a little and stretching your arms towards your feet. Breathe deeply, enjoying the aromas and the gentle stretch and release of tension in your back. Hold for 30 seconds.

04

Get out of the bath. Pat yourself dry and put on a robe.

05

Lie flat on your bed with no pillow for 15 minutes, allowing yourself time to fully feel the benefits of the ritual and to cool down, readying your body for sleep.

NEED TO KNOW

BENEFITS Eases muscle tension, especially in the back; helps you switch off at the end of the day.

TIME Around 30–50 minutes, in the evening.

PREPARATION If you wish, light candles and play calming music.

ITEMS REQUIRED **Massage oil:** Use the "Calming massage oil" blend (see pages 124–125). **Bath oil:** Add 2 drops each of the "Calming massage oil" essential oils to a warm bath.

RESTFUL SLEEP FACE MASSAGE

This gentle facial massage is an ideal opportunity for some relaxing "me-time" before you go to bed. The massage action unclenches your facial muscles and calms your cranial nerves, which in turn relaxes your whole body and quiets the mind. Practise every night as part of your preparation for a restful and restoring night's sleep.

NEED TO KNOW

BENEFITS Relaxes and tones facial muscles; calms body and mind before sleep; boosts circulation; reduces puffiness.

TIME 5–10 minutes nightly, at bedtime.

ITEMS NEEDED Your choice of facial oil blend (see pages 84–85).

01

Warm 2–3 drops of the massage oil in your palms. Cup your hands over your face and inhale through your nose to connect with the oil's aromas.

02

Apply the oil to your skin with long, sweeping movements from neck to forehead, avoiding the eyes.

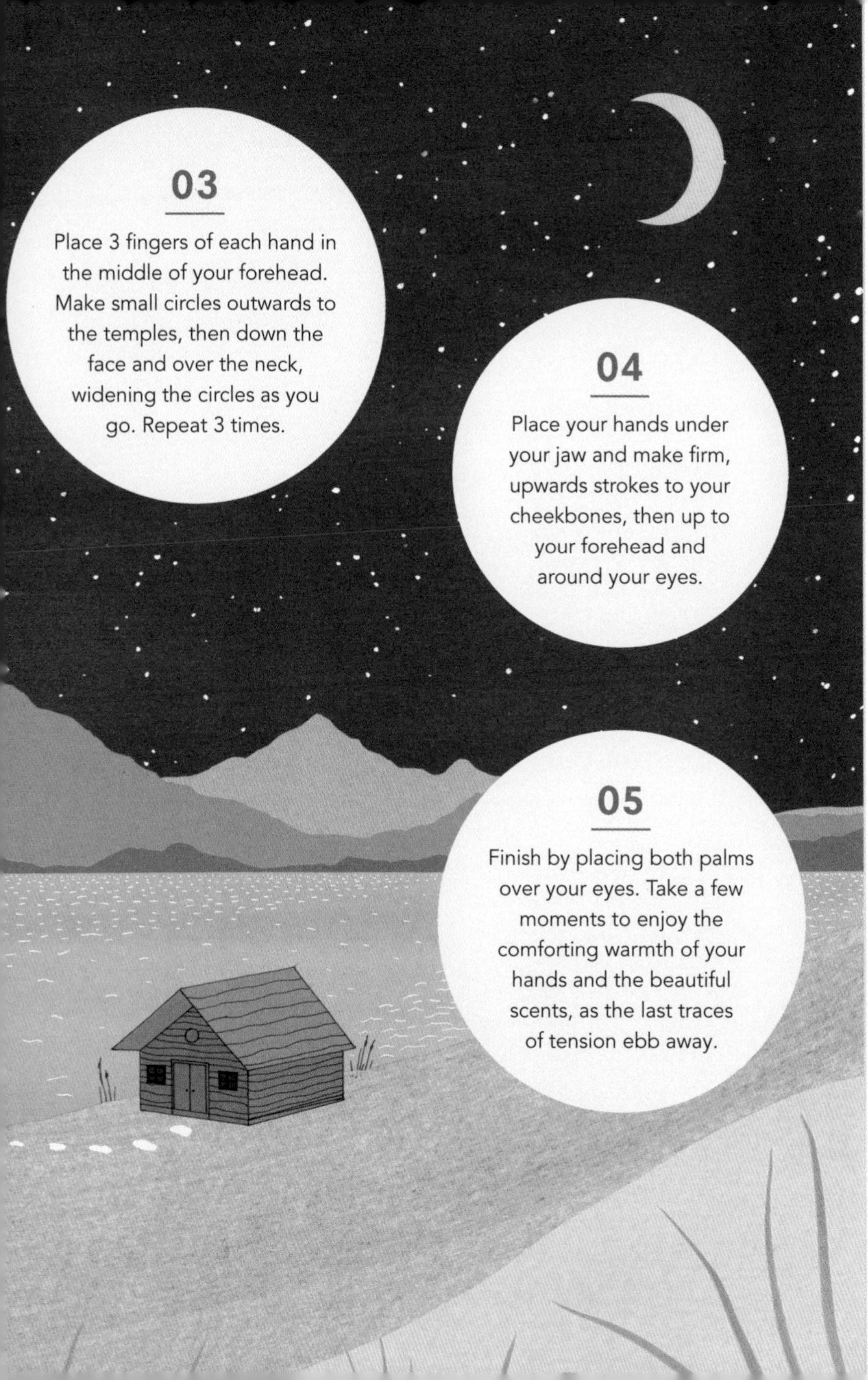

03

Place 3 fingers of each hand in the middle of your forehead. Make small circles outwards to the temples, then down the face and over the neck, widening the circles as you go. Repeat 3 times.

04

Place your hands under your jaw and make firm, upwards strokes to your cheekbones, then up to your forehead and around your eyes.

05

Finish by placing both palms over your eyes. Take a few moments to enjoy the comforting warmth of your hands and the beautiful scents, as the last traces of tension ebb away.

HEALING TREATMENTS

Essential oils are nature's first-aid kit – use them to provide immediate relief for cuts, grazes, and minor mishaps. They can also relieve symptoms of illness, reduce pain, and provide welcome support alongside medical treatment for serious or chronic conditions.

01

In a quiet place, put the essential oils on a tissue and hold it under your nose. Take slow nose breaths, savouring the grounding aroma.

02

Focus on an object near you, such as a lamp or a book. Concentrate only on the object and on your breathing. Now close your eyes.

03

Still concentrating on the object, slowly begin counting down from 10 to 1 in your head, repeating: "10, I am relaxing"... "9, I am relaxing...".

MANAGE OVERTHINKING

Constant thinking and ruminating can be distressing and exhausting. This simple, self-hypnosis exercise can help curb a too-busy mind – and essential oils enhance the practice through their grounding and clarifying properties.

04

Tell yourself that you are relaxing with every count and that, when you reach 1, you'll be in a peaceful, hypnotic state. Keep visualizing the object and focusing on your breaths.

05

Enjoy the calm for a few moments, then start to bring yourself back by counting up to 10, repeating, "1, my mind is calm"... "2, my mind is calm...". When you reach 10, inhale from the tissue again to feel alert and revived, and open your eyes.

NEED TO KNOW

BENEFITS Aids mental clarity, helping you to find a reflective response to worries and issues.

TIME 5–10 minutes at first, building up to 20–30 minutes as you become more practised.

ITEMS NEEDED Essential oils: 1 drop of vetiver, 2 drops each of lemon and frankincense; tissue.

SOOTHING, HEALING SKIN BLENDS

Essential oils can be used to soothe, heal, and treat a wide array of skin issues, from eczema and sunburn to chapped, sore, and itchy skin.

Your skin is your body's first line of defence against everything the world throws at it, and you can use aromatherapy to boost those defences. The essential oils in these blends have antibacterial, antimicrobial, anti-inflammatory, and antifungal properties. Have them to hand and you'll have your own natural first-aid kit for your skin.

BEST SKIN-SAVING ESSENTIAL OILS

Lavender	Lemon
Rose	German chamomile
Palmarosa	Roman chamomile
Myrrh	Tea tree
Frankincense	Patchouli

COLD COMPRESS FOR SUNBURN

The anti-inflammatory qualities of lavender and German chamomile cool, soothe and reduce the swelling of over-exposed skin. To use, soak a flannel in oil-infused water, wring it out, and apply to the affected area for about a minute. Repeat up to 3 times.

Makes 1 cold compress

Essential oils:

- 2 drops of German chamomile
- 3 drops of lavender

Other items:

Bowl of cold water; 1 tsp of grapeseed oil; cotton flannel

How to make

Combine the essential oils with the grapeseed oil, then add to the bowl of cold water.

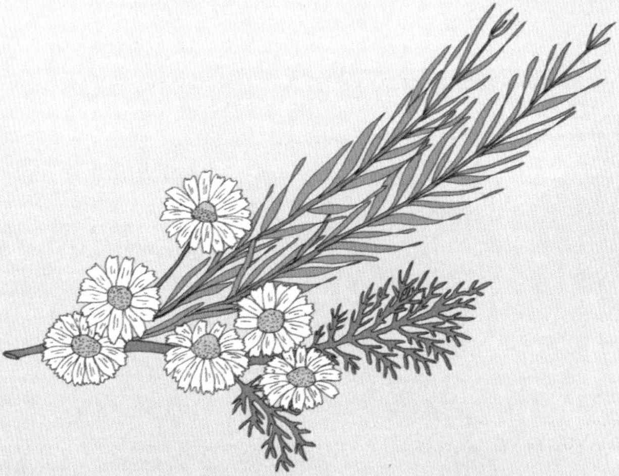

BALM FOR CUTS AND SCRATCHES

These oils have anti-inflammatory, antiseptic, and wound-healing qualities. Soothe chapped lips, insect bites, and sore or cut skin by rubbing into the affected area as needed.

Makes about 30g (1oz)

Essential oils:

- 2 drops of lavender
- 2 drops of Roman chamomile
- 2 drops of tea tree

Other items:

1 tsp of beeswax pellets; 1 tsp of shea butter; 1 tbsp of calendula macerated oil; heatproof glass bowl; small saucepan; mixing stick

How to make

To make the balm, follow the steps on pages 36–37.

SOOTHING CREAM

This blend can relieve the symptoms of eczema, psoriasis, and other dry skin conditions. To use, apply a thin layer to the affected area.

Makes 50g (1.8oz)

Essential oils:

- 5 drops of cedarwood atlas
- 5 drops of German chamomile
- 5 drops of lavender
- 5 drops of myrrh
- 5 drops of patchouli

Other items:

45g (1.6oz) of unfragranced organic cream base and 5g (0.2oz) of calendula macerated oil; small glass jar

How to make

Place the cream and calendula blend in the jar. Combine the essential oils, add to the cream and stir.

MANAGE COLDS AND COUGHS

Essential oils are ideal for fighting seasonal infections. They're versatile, too: use them as decongestants, chest rubs, and for steam inhalation.

The antimicrobial and immune-system stengthening qualities of some essential oils make them useful tools for fighting bugs and viruses. Eucalyptus is an effective decongestant and antiviral, while lavender and myrrh soothe cold and flu-like symptoms and will help you rest and reboot your system.

BEST ESSENTIAL OILS FOR COLDS

Black pepper	Myrrh
Pine	Cubeb
Eucalyptus	Lavender
Globulus	Cinnamon
Litsea	Cedarwood atlas

DECONGESTANT AROMASTICK

This blend will instantly clear blocked airways. In addition, the litsea and cinnamon are potent mood enhancers and immune-system stimulants.

Makes 1 aromastick

Essential oils:

- 1 drop of cinnamon
- 3 drops of eucalyptus radiata
- 3 drops of litsea
- 3 drops of pine

Other items:

Aromastick

How to make

Add the essential oils to the aromastick. Inhale throughout the day as required.

EVENING STEAM INHALATION

If you have a troublesome cough, try this inhalation about half an hour before you go to bed. It will open your airways and release congestion to promote a good night's sleep. Cover your head and the bowl with a towel and inhale the steam for 5–10 minutes.

Makes 1 steam inhalation

Essential oils:

- 2 drops of cedarwood atlas
- 2 drops of lavender
- 2 drops of myrrh

Other items:

Bowl of water; towel

How to make

Sprinkle the essential oils onto a bowl of just-boiled water.

WARMING BATH OIL

This blend will relieve aches and pains, unblock a congested nose, and clear your fuzzy head.

Makes 1 bath blend

Essential oils:

- 3 drops of bergamot
- 3 drops of black pepper
- 4 drops of lavender

Other items:

20ml (0.7fl oz) of almond oil, milk, or unfragranced bath foamer base

How to make

Mix the essential oils with your chosen base and add to a warm bath.

BLENDS FOR NAUSEA AND INDIGESTION

Inhaling certain essential oils can quickly quell feelings of nausea and indigestion, while applying them directly can help to calm an upset stomach.

Nausea and gastric upsets can be caused by a variety of things, including rich, spicy, or contaminated food, migraine, or travel sickness, but these issues can often be settled quickly by the right combination of essential oils. The blends here are designed to settle feelings of queasiness, and have muscle-relaxing and pain-relieving properties, too.

BEST ESSENTIAL OILS FOR DIGESTION

Sweet orange	Cardamom
Grapefruit	Coriander
Ginger	Lavender
Peppermint	Lemon

NAUSEA-CALMING AROMASTICK

Inhaling zesty and warming lemon and ginger can quickly settle your system and ease feelings of nausea.

Makes 1 aromastick

Essential oils:

- 5 drops of ginger
- 5 drops of lemon

Other items:

Aromastick

How to make

Add essential oils to your aromastick (see pages 44–45). Inhale as required.

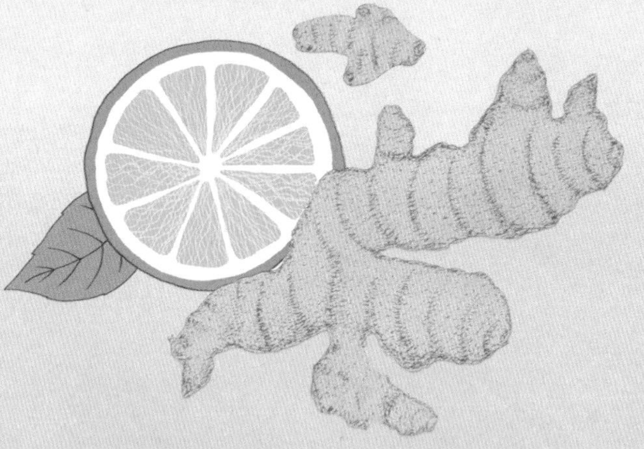

WARMING STOMACH COMPRESS

Use this compress to relieve cramps and pains. The sweet orange and coriander will also soothe your digestion.

Makes 1 warm compress

Essential oils:

- 3 drops of coriander
- 3 drops of sweet orange

Other items:

Cotton flannel; warm water;
1 tsp of grapeseed oil

How to make

Combine the essential oils with the grapeseed oil, then add to a bowl of warm water. Soak the flannel in the water, wring it out and lay it across the stomach for about a minute. Repeat up to 3 times.

ANTI-BLOATING MASSAGE

For bloating and cramping, try a soothing massage (see pages 102–103) with this blend. If you have sensitive skin, patch test the peppermint before use (see pages 22–23).

Makes 30ml (1fl oz)

Essential oils:

- 3 drops of peppermint
- 6 drops of sweet marjoram
- 6 drops of sweet orange

Other items:

30ml (1fl oz) of grapeseed oil;
small bottle with lid

How to make

Pour the grapeseed oil into the bottle then add the essential oils. Put the lid on and shake to combine.

01

Lie on your back with knees bent and a pillow under your head.

02

Warm 3–4 drops of the massage oil in your palms. Cup your hands over your face and inhale the clean, reviving aroma.

03

Put the palm of one hand over your belly button. Slowly and gently massage the skin in a clockwise direction. This encourages a sluggish digestive system to push food through your gut.

SOOTHING ABDOMINAL MASSAGE

Painful abdominal bloating and spasms can be stress-related, as well as symptoms of IBS (irritable bowel syndrome). This massage relieves pain and encourages sluggish digestion to reduce bloating. The essential oils are especially effective for flare-ups triggered by anxiety.

05

Finish by resting both hands on your abdomen. Take a few minutes to tune in to how your body is feeling while your skin absorbs the oils fully.

04

Continue the slow, gentle movement for about 5 minutes, gradually widening the area and applying a little more pressure – ease off if this causes discomfort.

NEED TO KNOW

BENEFITS Warms and relaxes tense, cramping gut muscles; calms the mind and nervous system.

TIME 5–10 minutes. Perform as often as needed.

PREPARATION Make up the "Anti-bloating massage" blend on pages 100–101.

MASSAGE AWAY HEADACHES

Essential oils, combined with massage, are an excellent way to treat headaches of all types. Lavender and peppermint make a simple and effective combination to relieve pain and melt away tension.

NEED TO KNOW

BENEFITS Cools body and mind and breaks the cycle of tension that causes head pain, which leads to more muscle tension and greater pain.

TIME 5–10 minutes, as needed.

ITEMS NEEDED 2 drops of peppermint and 4 drops of lavender essential oils, blended with 30ml (1fl oz) of grapeseed oil.

PREPARATION In a quiet place, sit comfortably on an upright chair in front of a table.

01

Warm 2–3 drops of the massage oil in your palms. Cup your hands over your face and inhale slowly and deeply, feeling the soothing, cooling aroma start to relieve the tension in your head.

02

Place your index and middle fingers on each temple and gently massage the area with small, circular motions.

03

Rest your elbows on the table. Close your eyes, placing the heel of each hand over your eyes. Hold for a count of 10, breathing deeply. Repeat steps 2 and 3 as required, until your head clears.

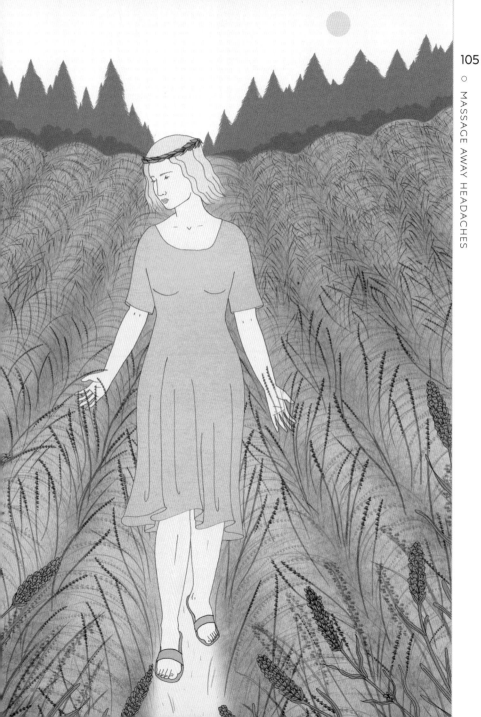

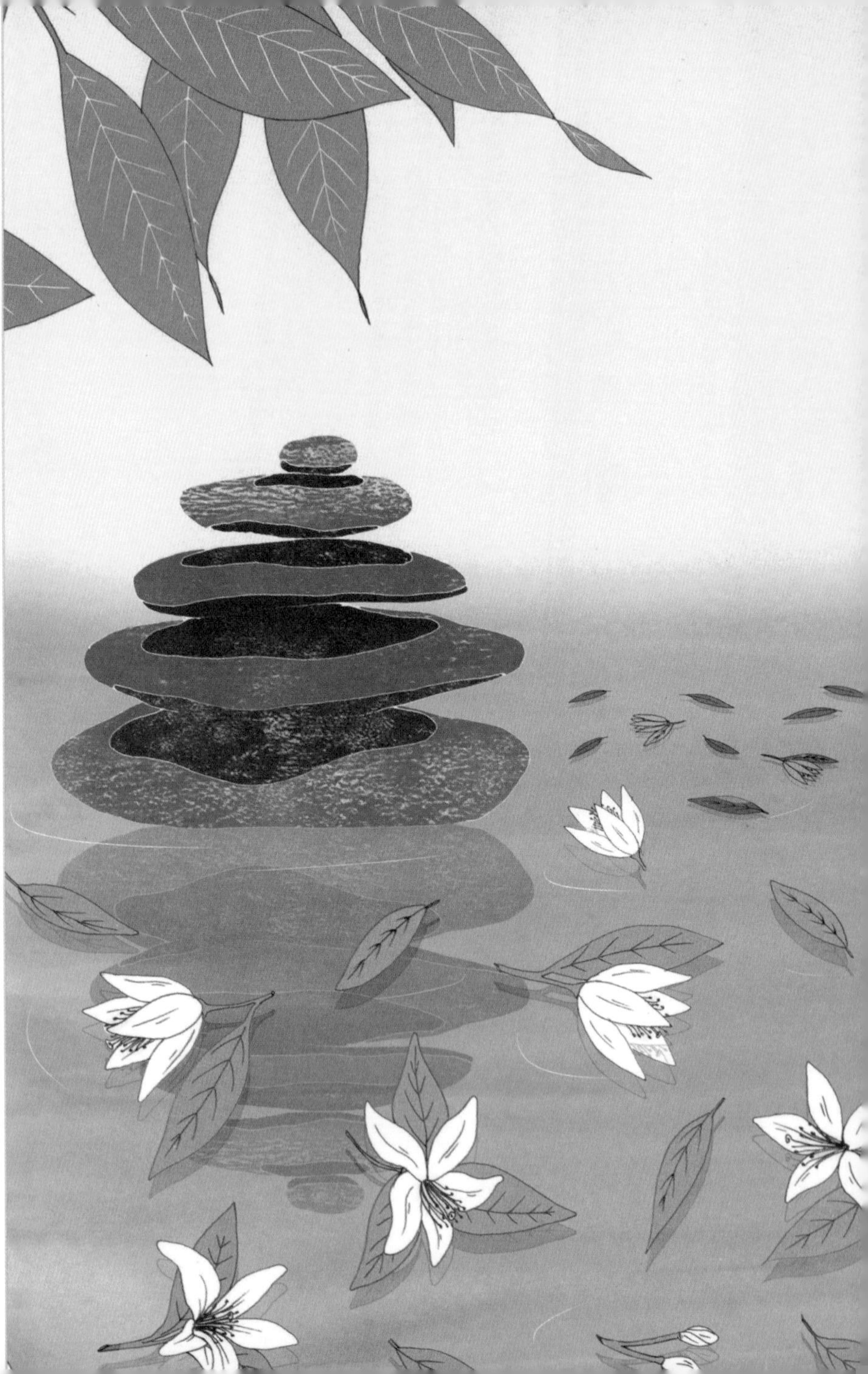

EMERGENCY RESCUE BLEND

If you've had a shock, or feel panicky about an upcoming stressful event, this blend makes a powerful SOS remedy. Neroli calms the heart and the nervous system, so is perfect for acute situations.

BENEFITS Quickly eases feelings of shock and panic; helps restore emotional balance.

TIME 5 minutes, as often as required.

ITEMS NEEDED Essential oils: 1 drop of Roman chamomile, 2 drops each of neroli and petitgrain; 10ml (0.35fl oz) of sunflower oil; glass rollette bottle.

PREPARATION Add the sunflower oil and the essential oils to the rollette bottle and shake to combine.

01

For the quickest relief, use the rescue blend on your main pulse points (see page 38). Begin by rolling a small amount over the radial pulse points on your wrists.

02

Then roll the blend over your carotid (neck) pulse points. Next, apply it to both temporal pulse points, on your temples.

03

Finally, roll a little oil onto both palms, cup your hands over your face, and inhale the calming aroma of the oils. Continue until your breathing is steady.

SKIN FIRST-AID REMEDIES

When stocking up your first-aid kit, make sure it includes some essential oil remedies like these to help cut, grazed, and inflamed skin heal quickly and naturally.

Essential oils are versatile and should be vital components of your natural first-aid kit. The oils in these blends are especially effective for treating the skin; as well as being naturally antibacterial, antifungal, and antimicrobial, they also reduce inflammation and relieve pain.

BEST SKIN-REPAIR ESSENTIAL OILS

Lavender	Patchouli
Myrrh	Petitgrain
Frankincense	Yarrow
Rose	Roman chamomile
Tea tree	German chamomile

BITES AND RASHES COMPRESS

The antibacterial and anti-allergenic qualities of this blend will reduce the itchiness of insect bites and hives. To use, soak the flannel in the oil-infused water, wring it out and apply to the affected skin for a few minutes. Repeat up to 3 times.

Makes 1 cold compress

Essential oils:

- 1 drop of lavender
- 1 drop of thyme
- 2 drops of German chamomile

Other items:

Cotton flannel; bowl; 1 tsp of grapeseed oil

How to make

Fill the bowl with cold water. Combine the essential oils with the grapeseed oil, then add to the water.

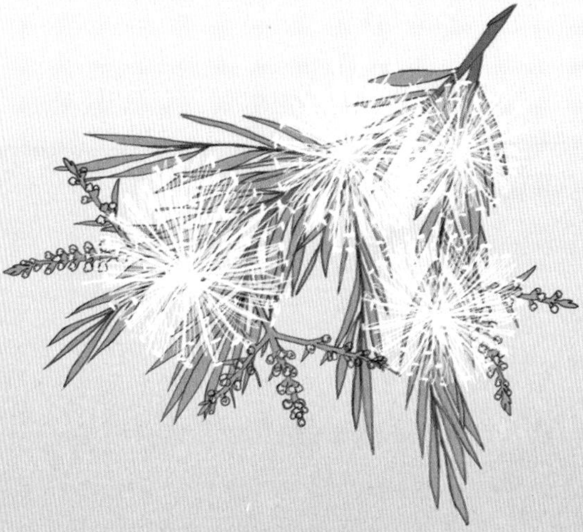

ATHLETE'S FOOT GEL

Apply this healing, antifungal gel to clean, dry feet to soothe the sore, itchy skin that comes with athlete's foot.

Makes 50ml (1.75fl oz) of gel

Essential oils:

- 3 drops of myrrh
- 3 drops of tea tree
- 4 drops of lavender

Other items:

50ml (1.75fl oz) of aloe vera gel; small jar with lid

How to make

Place the gel in a jar. Add the essential oils and stir to combine. Apply a thin layer to the affected skin and leave to soak in before putting on footwear.

BLISTER BLITZER

Treat blisters quickly and easily with this remedy, which both soothes and speeds up the healing process.

Makes 1 treatment

Essential oils:

- 1 drop of lavender

Other items:

Cold, wet, used teabag (black or green tea)

How to make

Add the lavender to the teabag and place it over the blister for about 5 minutes. The tannin in the tea reduces swelling while the lavender provides pain relief and heals the skin.

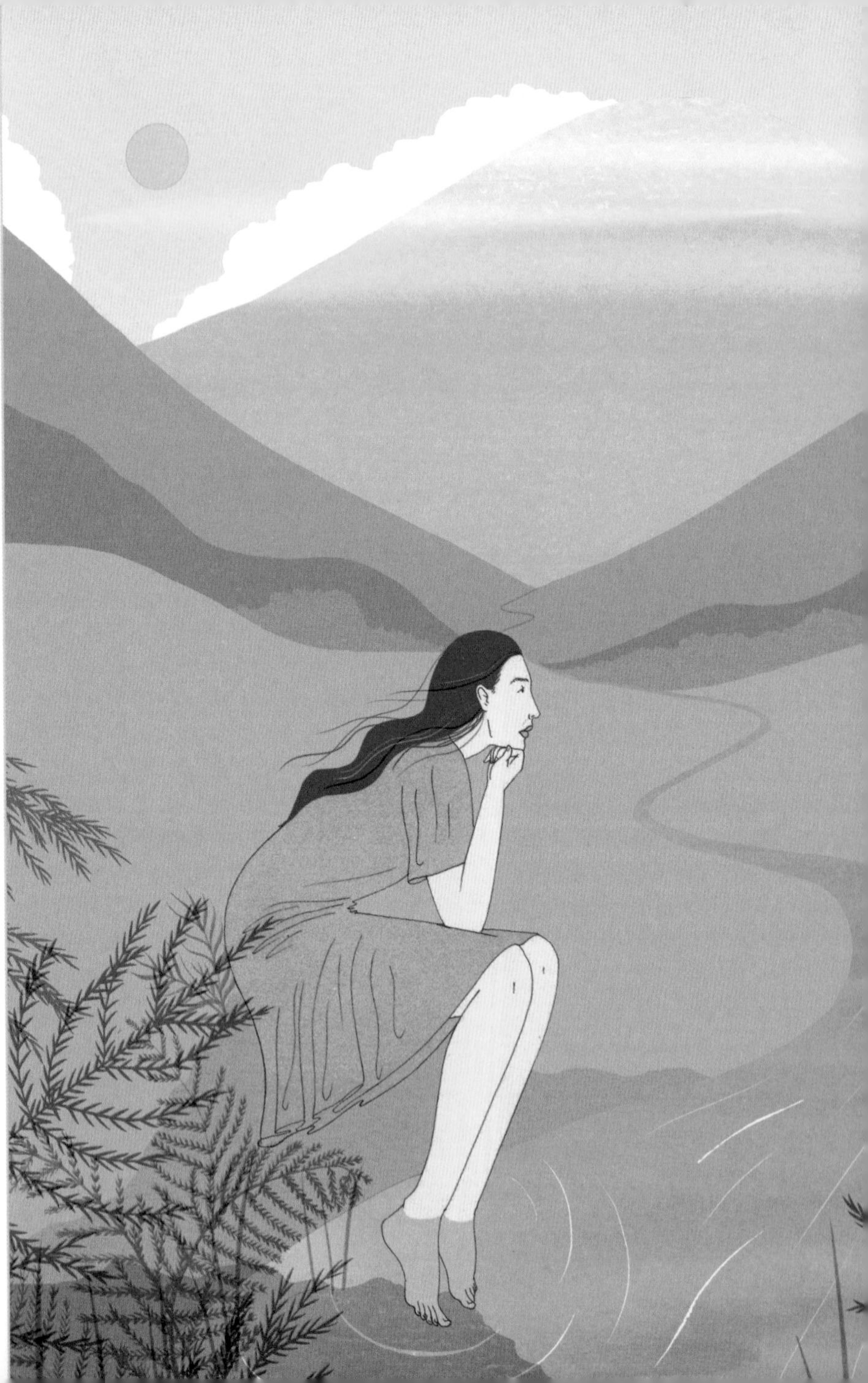

FATIGUE-RELIEVING FOOT SOAK

At the end of a long, tiring day, restore yourself from your toes up with this foot soak, which combines refreshing, soothing oils of peppermint, lavender, and lemon with Epsom salts to relieve aches and pains.

NEED TO KNOW

BENEFITS Refreshes tired, aching feet; Epsom salts draw toxins from the body.

TIME About 15 minutes, in the evening or as required.

PREPARATION Fill a bowl with warm water. Add 1 tbsp of Epsom salts and 2 drops each of lavender, lemon, and peppermint essential oils.

01

Before you put your feet in the bowl, gently rub each foot for a few minutes. This releases tension and softens the skin, readying it to absorb the essential oils.

02

Place your feet in the bowl and let them soak for around 10 minutes. While you enjoy the soothing sensations, breathe deeply and slowly, taking in the oils' reviving aroma.

03

Dry your feet thoroughly and finish by gently rubbing them with a massage oil of your choice, or use the "Relaxing massage oil" blend on pages 112–113.

RELIEF FOR MUSCLE ACHES AND PAINS

Essential oils are nature's power house when it comes to treating pain and discomfort. These blends are specially designed to work on sore, tight, and overworked muscles, helping them to relax, recuperate, and repair themselves.

The healing powers of essential oils don't only come from inhaling their scent – we can also absorb their active ingredients through the skin, straight into the bloodstream. This means that their anti-inflammatory, analgesic properties can be delivered straight to your muscles and joints, to reduce swelling, relieve tightness, and ease pain.

BEST ESSENTIAL OILS FOR MUSCLES

Lemongrass	Black pepper
Lavandin	Sweet marjoram
Plai	Rosemary
Bay laurel	Cardamom
Ginger	Lavender

SPORTY SHOWER GEL

Refresh and invigorate tired post-workout muscles with this shower gel enhanced with warming black pepper and stimulating lemongrass.

Makes 100ml (3.5fl oz)

Essential oils:

- 10 drops of black pepper
- 10 drops of cardamom
- 10 drops of lemongrass
- 15 drops of lavandin

Other items:

100ml (3.5fl oz) of unfragranced shower gel; small plastic bottle with lid

How to make

Add the essential oils and the shower gel to the bottle and shake to combine. Use as necessary.

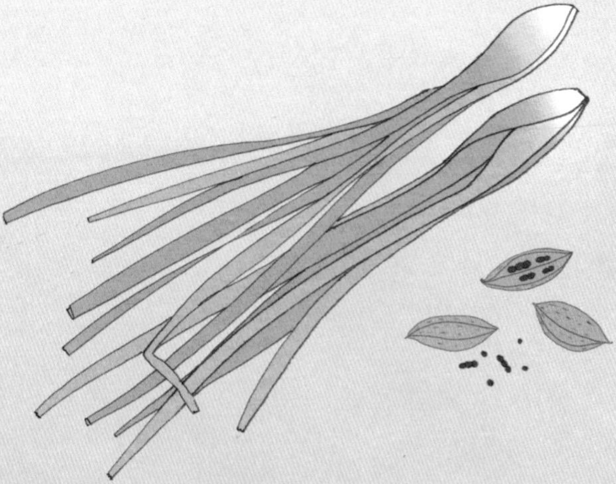

SOOTHING BATH BLEND

Soak away aches and pains with this comforting bath blend. The essential oils here have pain-relieving and anti-inflammatory qualities.

Makes 1 bath blend

Essential oils:

- 3 drops of coriander
- 3 drops of sweet marjoram
- 4 drops of lavender

Other items:

20ml (0.7fl oz) of almond oil or unfragranced bath foamer base

How to make

Mix the essential oils with your chosen base and add to a warm bath.

RELAXING MASSAGE OIL

Use this blend on tired, painful muscles to relieve tension and promote restful sleep. In addition, the arnica reduces inflammation.

Makes 30ml (1fl oz)

Essential oils:

- 3 drops of cardamom
- 3 drops of plai
- 4 drops of lavender
- 5 drops of frankincense

Other items:

30ml (1fl oz) of arnica macerated oil; small plastic bottle with lid

How to make

Pour the oil into the bottle then add the essential oils. Put the lid on and shake to combine. To perform a massage, follow the steps on pages 130–131.

HELP FOR PAINFUL JOINTS

You can treat aching joints with a daily self-massage or compress, both using healing, nourishing, and warming essential oils. As well as relieving pain and inflammation, they will stimulate the circulation, pumping more oxygen into the blood to speed the healing process.

DAILY MASSAGE OIL

Gently rub this anti-inflammatory blend in to achy joints to aid mobility and boost blood circulation.

Makes 30ml (1fl oz)

Essential oils:

- 1 drop of cinnamon
- 4 drops of bay laurel
- 4 drops of lemon eucalyptus
- 4 drops of plai

Other items:

30ml (1fl oz) of arnica macerated oil; small plastic bottle with lid

How to make

Pour the arnica oil into the bottle then add the essential oils. Put the lid on and shake to combine.

JOINT-COOLING COMPRESS

When joints are very painful, massage may not be helpful. Try this gentle cold compress blend instead. Soak the flannel, wring it out and place it on the affected area for 1 minute. Repeat up to 3 times.

Makes 1 cold compress

Essential oils:

- 2 drops of German chamomile
- 3 drops of lavandin

Other items:

A bowl of cold water and a flannel; 1 tsp grapeseed oil

How to make

Combine the essential oils with the grapeseed oil and add to the bowl of water.

BEST ESSENTIAL OILS FOR JOINTS

- Niaouli
- Lavandin
- Bay laurel
- Ginger
- Black pepper
- German chamomile
- Thyme
- Cinnamon
- Lemon eucalyptus
- Plai

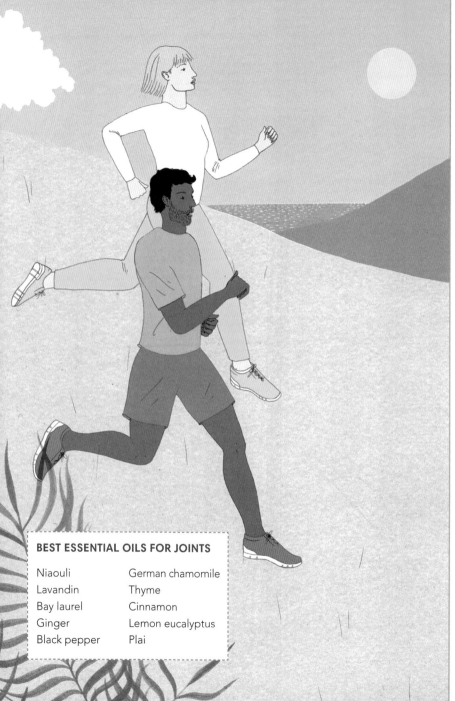

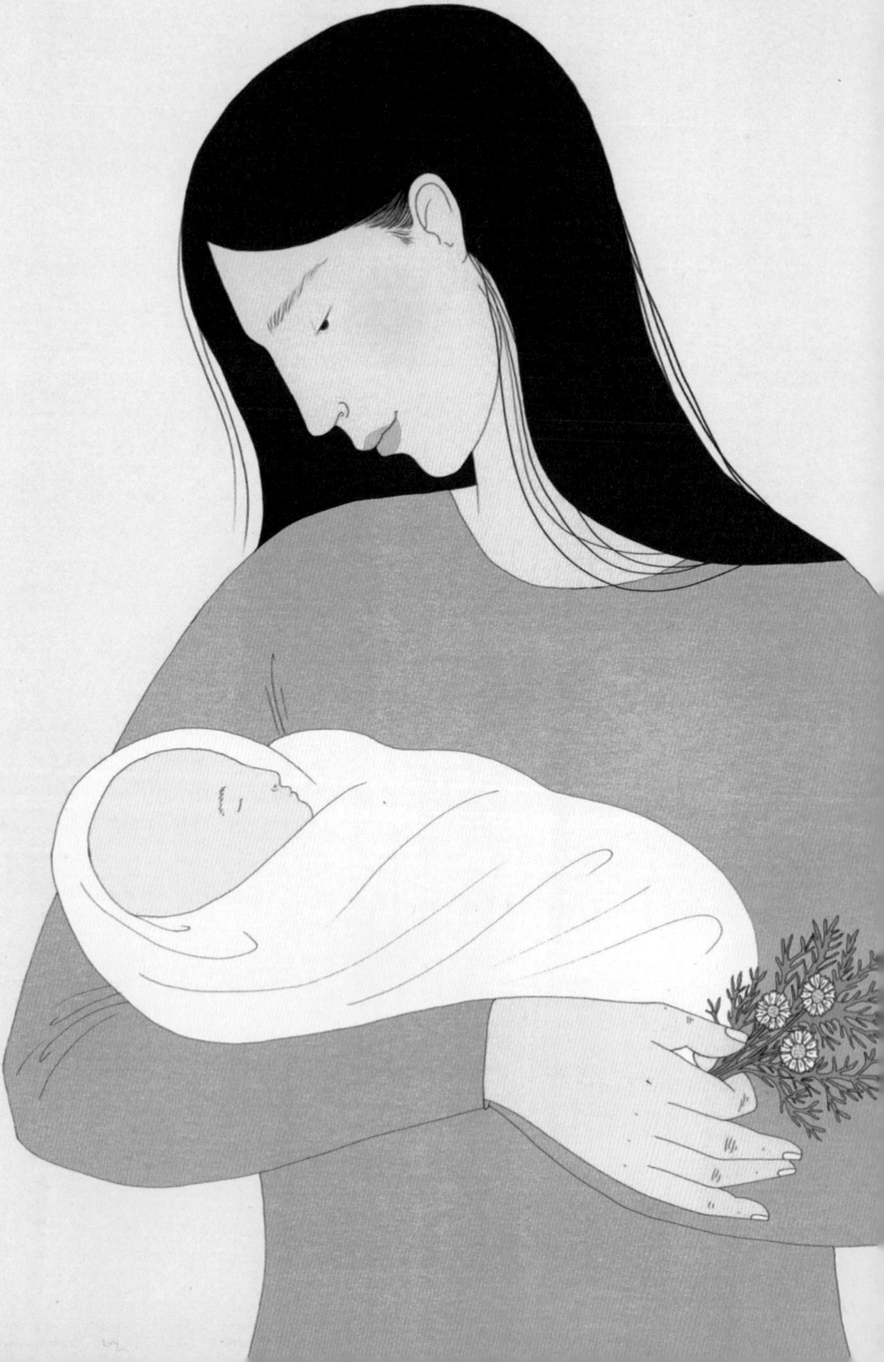

HEALING POST-NATAL HIP BATH

After childbirth there is a period of physical recovery for new mothers. An essential oil-infused hip bath, also called a sitz bath, is an age-old remedy, which will both speed the healing process and help you regain your energy.

NEED TO KNOW

BENEFITS Relieves pain and aids healing of tears and episiotomy stitches.

TIME 5–10 minutes. Bathe 3 times a day at first, then less frequently as you heal.

ITEMS NEEDED
For 1 bath: 2 drops each of lavender, Roman chamomile and tea tree essential oils mixed with 30ml (1fl oz) of macerated calendula oil.

01

Fill a bath or baby bath with warm water to hip height, or around 20–25cm (8–10in). Make up the blend, add it to the bath, and allow it to disperse.

02

Lower yourself into the bath and soak for 5–10 minutes, letting the healing oils take effect while you breathe in their reviving aromas.

03

Take care getting out of the bath as it will be slippery. Dry yourself gently and thoroughly, checking the progress of any wounds or sore areas.

MANAGING MENSTRUAL ISSUES

There is a range of essential oils to call on that offer a natural way for you to manage the hormone-driven ups and downs of your monthly menstrual cycle.

These blends are designed to balance your hormones and calm symptoms such as heavy and painful periods and mood swings. It may take at least two months or more for you to feel the full benefit of these remedies, so stick with them.

Every woman will respond to essential oils differently, so experiment with the other oils listed below to find the best blend for you.

BEST HORMONE-BALANCING ESSENTIAL OILS

Rose	Fennel
Cypress	Clary sage
Sweet marjoram	Lavender
Geranium	Peppermint
Aniseed	Neroli

INHALATION FOR PMT

Use this if you are feeling irritable, moody, or just discombobulated! All these oils will help to reset your hormones and lift your spirit.

Makes 1 inhalation

Essential oils:

- 3 drops of cypress
- 3 drops of geranium
- 4 drops of bergamot

Other items:

Tissue or aromastick

How to make

Add the essential oils to a tissue or aromastick. Use throughout the day as required.

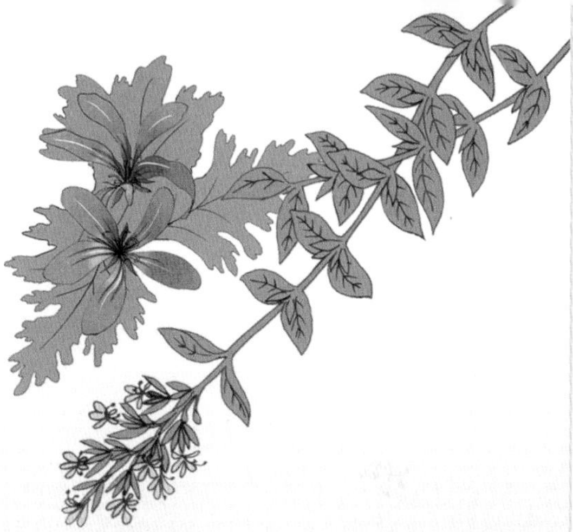

BALANCING BATH BLEND

When you've been feeling out of sorts all day, soothe yourself with this bath blend to restore equilibrium and ensure a good night's sleep.

Makes 1 bath blend

Essential oils:

- 2 drops of geranium
- 2 drops of rose
- 3 drops of lavender
- 3 drops of sweet marjoram

Other items:

20ml (0.7fl oz) of almond oil or unfragranced bath foamer base

How to make

Mix the essential oils with your chosen base and add to a warm bath.

PAINFUL PERIODS MASSAGE OIL

This blend's essential oils help to settle hormones, ease cramping, and reduce pain. When you feel your period starting, massage the oil over your abdomen, lower back, and thighs. Perform morning and evening for the duration of your period.

Makes 30ml (1fl oz)

Essential oils:

- 3 drops of clary sage
- 3 drops of fennel
- 3 drops of sweet marjoram
- 4 drops of rose

Other items:

30ml (1fl oz) of grapeseed oil; small plastic bottle with lid

How to make

Pour the grapeseed oil into the bottle and add the essential oils. Put the lid on and shake to combine.

TREATING MENOPAUSE SYMPTOMS

Menopause is a time of profound hormonal change in every woman's life. Alongside a healthy lifestyle, aromatherapy can play a key role in tackling the challenges and changes you may face.

Every woman's menopause is different, but making up natural treatments and having them to hand can help you feel better prepared to cope with symptoms that might arise, such as hot flushes, night sweats, palpitations, anxiety, and depression. The essential oils in these blends help to dial down symptoms by balancing hormones, calming anxiety, relaxing muscles, easing cramps, and boosting mood.

BEST MENOPAUSE ESSENTIAL OILS

Rose	Fennel
Geranium	Sweet marjoram
Cypress	Cardamom
Clary sage	Palmarosa
Spanish sage	Basil

MOOD-BOOSTER AROMASTICK

Instantly quell irritability, anxiety, or depression and feel sharper, soothed, and in balance with this uplifting inhalation blend.

Makes 1 aromastick

Essential oils:

- 2 drops of basil
- 2 drops of bergamot
- 2 drops of rosemary
- 4 drops of geranium

Other items:

Aromastick

How to make

Add the essential oils to the aromastick. Inhale throughout the day as required.

COOLING SPRITZ

Hot flushes start when blood vessels close to the skin's surface widen to cool off, making you sweat. Whenever a hot flush strikes, spritz this cooling blend once or twice on your chest and abdomen.

Makes 100ml (3.5fl oz)

Essential oils:

- 3 drops of clary sage
- 3 drops of cypress
- 4 drops of geranium

Other items:

100ml (3.5fl oz) of rose water or plain water; spritz bottle

How to make

Pour the water into the bottle and add the essential oils. Screw on the bottle's nozzle and shake to combine before every use.

HORMONE-BALANCING OIL

Rub in a little of this all-over body oil every day to address hormone imbalance and alleviate symptoms. Avoid using this blend on your face.

Makes 30ml (1fl oz)

Essential oils:

- 3 drops of bergamot
- 3 drops of black spruce
- 3 drops of fennel
- 6 drops of geranium

Other items:

30ml (1fl oz) of grapeseed oil; small plastic bottle with lid

How to make

Pour the grapeseed oil into the bottle then add the essential oils. Put the lid on and shake to combine.

ANGER-CALMING RITUAL

Inhaling calming bergamot essential oil as you practise a body relaxation technique is a quick and effective way to quell anger and restore your good temper. Use it whenever you feel work pressures, stress, or the irritations and frustrations of daily life getting the better of you.

01

Close your eyes and hold the oil-infused tissue under your nose. Inhale slowly and deeply, fully engaging with the fresh, bright aroma.

NEED TO KNOW

BENEFITS Immediately reduces the physical and psychological effects of anger. Calms the nervous system and restores emotional equilibrium.

TIME About 20 minutes, as required.

PREPARATION Find a quiet place and lie down on the floor or a firm bed.

ITEMS NEEDED
A tissue doused with a few drops of bergamot essential oil.

02

Place the tissue on your chest. Relax and try to let your mind drift. Be conscious of your breath as you continue to breathe slowly and deeply.

03

Slowly, tense all the muscles in your feet. Hold for a few seconds, then relax. Repeat for your calves, thighs, buttocks, stomach, arms, hands, shoulders, and face, all the time breathing deeply and consciously.

04

Now bring the tissue back up to your face again and lie quietly for 10–15 minutes, inhaling deeply and allowing any remaining negative feelings to subside.

BLENDS TO LIFT A LOW MOOD

Use the power of aromatherapy to clear the grey skies in your heart and mind, and give you a much-needed lift when times are tough.

Life continuously throws us challenges that can knock us back. Apart from work, relationship, or family worries, even a happy event like having a baby brings its share of low moments, too. When you're struggling to feel the joy, you may lose your appetite or turn to food for comfort; your sleep might be disrupted and your energy level is stuck at zero. The therapeutic properties of essential oils can raise flagging spirits and help you feel ready to face the world again.

BEST UPLIFTING ESSENTIAL OILS

Rose	Melissa
Geranium	Sweet orange
Cypress	Ylang ylang
Clary sage	Mandarin
Bergamot	Basil

INSTANT SUNSHINE INHALATION

This blend will immediately make you feel as if the clouds have cleared to reveal the sun. The melissa in particular will give you clarity and relieve emotional lows and mental pressures.

Makes 1 tissue inhalation

Essential oils:

- 2 drops of black spruce
- 3 drops of melissa
- 4 drops of bergamot

Other items:

Tissue; small plastic bag

How to make

Add the essential oil drops to the tissue and inhale. Put the tissue in the bag to carry with you and use as needed.

CALMING MASSAGE OIL

Use this blend to quieten your nervous system and help you cope with challenging feelings. Lie down and massage using clockwise strokes on your solar plexus, just below your chest, for a few minutes.

Makes 1 massage blend

Essential oils:

- 3 drops of basil
- 3 drops of mandarin
- 4 drops of neroli
- 4 drops of cypress

Other items:

30ml (1fl oz) of grapeseed oil; small plastic bottle with lid

How to make

Pour the grapeseed oil into the bottle then add the essential oils. Put the lid on and shake to combine.

UPLIFTING AROMASTICK

The essential oils geranium and clary sage are excellent mood improvers, and are especially helpful for resetting fluctuating, post-childbirth hormones.

Makes 1 aromastick

Essential oils:

- 2 drops of clary sage
- 2 drops of lavender
- 2 drops of sweet orange
- 4 drops of geranium

Other items:

Aromastick

How to make

Add the essential oils to the aromastick. Inhale as needed.

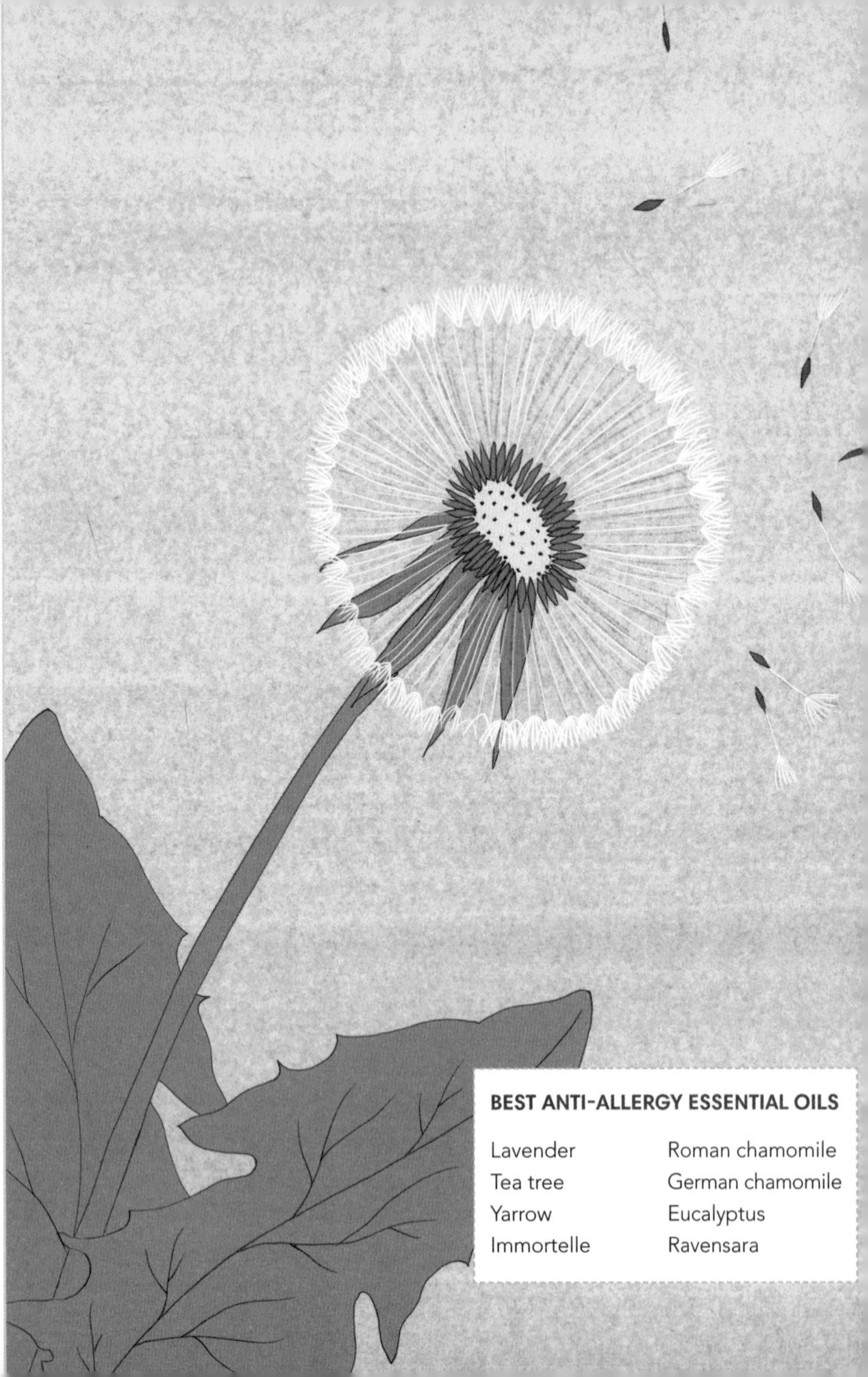

BEST ANTI-ALLERGY ESSENTIAL OILS

Lavender	Roman chamomile
Tea tree	German chamomile
Yarrow	Eucalyptus
Immortelle	Ravensara

ALLERGY ANTIDOTES

Allergic reactions – the sign that our bodies are working overtime to protect us from invaders such as dust, pollen, or animal hair – are annoyingly common. The good news is that essential-oil compresses and balms can help to alleviate many of the uncomfortable symptoms of allergies.

COOLING COMPRESS

This blend of anti-inflammatory and antiseptic oils will soothe an allergic rash. To use, soak the flannel in the oil-infused water, wring it out and apply it to the affected area until it cools. Repeat up to 3 times. For a more widespread rash, add the oils in the same proportions to a warm bath.

Makes 1 cold compress

Essential oils:

- 1 drop of German chamomile
- 1 drop of yarrow
- 3 drops of lavender

Other items:

Cotton flannel; bowl of cold water; 1 tsp of grapeseed oil

How to make

Combine the oils and add them to the water.

HAY FEVER BALM

Dab this around your nostrils and on your cheeks, to act as a barrier to dust and pollen, soothe sore skin, and stop eyes feeling itchy and watery.

Makes about 30ml (1fl oz)

Essential oils:

- 2 drops of Roman chamomile
- 4 drops of lavender

Other items:

1 tbsp of calendula macerated oil; 1 tsp each of beeswax pellets and shea butter; heatproof glass bowl; small saucepan; mixing stick

How to make

See pages 36–37 for how to make a balm.

COPING WITH ANXIETY

Because aromatherapy and essential oils work holistically on the mind, body, and spirit, they can provide vital support for conditions that affect us both physically and mentally, such as anxiety.

Some anxiety is a natural response to stress, but heightened or prolonged levels can wreak havoc on our health. Use essential oils to treat mild anxiety yourself, or as an add-on to ongoing medical treatment. These three blends will all help to dial down panic; each contains at least one essential oil with proven calming properties. If you mix your own blend to include a favourite scent, make sure you use at least one of the proven worry-busters listed below.

BEST ESSENTIAL OILS FOR ANXIETY

Mandarin	Lemon
Frankincense	Cypress
Lavender	Vetiver
Patchouli	Roman chamomile
Bergamot	Clary sage

LAVENDER PATCHOULI DIFFUSION

Use this rich, spicy blend in a room diffuser to create a calming environment in the home or workplace.

Makes 1 diffusion

Essential oils:

- 2 drops of lavender
- 2 drops of patchouli

Other items:

Room diffuser

How to make

Add the recommended amount of water to the diffuser then add the drops of essential oils to the surface.

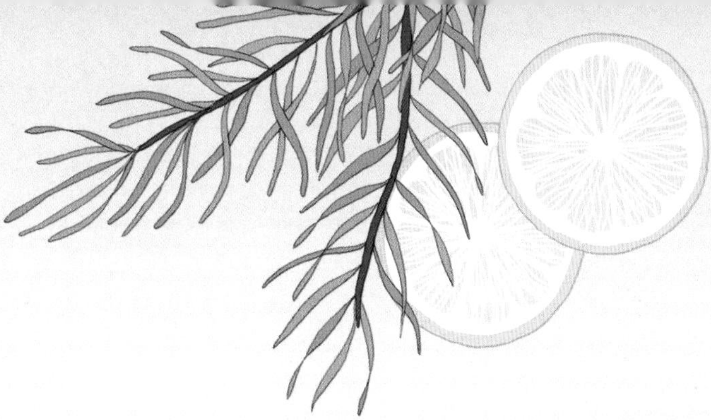

BEDTIME MASSAGE OIL

If worries keep you awake at night, gently massage this blend into your chest and neck before bed.

Makes 30ml (1fl oz)

Essential oils:

- 3 drops of vetiver
- 6 drops of frankincense
- 6 drops of lavender

Other items:

30ml (1fl oz) of grapeseed oil; small plastic bottle, with lid

How to make

Pour the grapeseed oil into the bottle, then add the essential oils. Place the lid on and shake to mix together.

FIRST-AID INHALATION

This blend makes a great SOS remedy – a few drops on a tissue provides an instant antidote to mounting anxiety.

Makes 1 tissue inhalation

Essential oils:

- 1 drop of bergamot
- 1 drop of cypress
- 1 drop of lemon

Other items:

Tissue; small plastic bag

How to make

Add the essential oil drops to a folded tissue and inhale. Put the tissue in the bag to carry with you and use as needed.

01

Sit comfortably and warm a few drops of massage oil in your palms by rubbing them together.

02

Begin by massaging the top, bottom, and toes of your right foot, then your lower leg. Rub behind the knee to stimulate the lymphatic system, then massage the upper leg and buttocks. Repeat on your other leg.

POST-ILLNESS REVITALIZING MASSAGE

Recovering from a virus or cold can leave you feeling drained. This self-massage stimulates and tones your skin and muscles, helping you to regain your vitality. Use slow, gentle strokes for this exercise.

03

Using the flat of one palm, massage your abdomen gently in a clockwise direction. Move up to the chest and sweep down each arm several times.

04

With the fingertips of both hands, gently massage your neck, then use broad, gentle strokes with both palms to brush your shoulders and upper back 3 or 4 times.

05

When you've finished, cover up and stay warm. If you can, allow 12 hours before showering so that the oils can be absorbed fully into your body.

NEED TO KNOW

BENEFITS Relaxes aches and pains; boosts blood and lymphatic circulation.

TIME 10–15 minutes, as needed.

ITEMS NEEDED Use the "Immunity-boosting massage" blend on pages 62–63 for this exercise, or a blend of your choice.

HANDY TRAVEL REMEDIES

The next time you take a trip, bring your own mobile pharmacy with you. These two versatile blends comprise an essential traveller's first-aid kit, designed to tackle the ill effects of too much sun, nausea, and irritating insects.

TRAVEL-SICKNESS BLEND

These essential oils are fantastic for subduing nausea. Using them in an aromastick creates a discreet treatment you can take anywhere.

Makes 1 aromastick

Essential oils:

- 3 drops of ginger
- 3 drops of peppermint
- 4 drops of lemon

Other items:

Aromastick

How to make

Add the essential oils to the aromastick. Inhale as needed.

ALL-PURPOSE HOLIDAY LOTION

The essential oils in this blend treat heat exhaustion, sunburn, and insect bites; calendula nourishes and heals the skin, while neem oil repels bugs.

Makes 250ml (9fl oz)

Essential oils:

- 6 drops of eucalyptus
- 6 drops of Roman chamomile
- 6 drops of thyme linalool
- 8 drops of lavender

Other items:

5ml (0.17fl oz) neem oil; 10ml (0.35fl oz) calendula macerated oil; 235ml (8.3fl oz) unfragranced lotion; plastic bottle with lid

How to make

Pour the lotion and all the oils into the bottle and shake to combine. Use on clean, dry skin, avoiding the face.

BEST TRAVEL ESSENTIAL OILS

Lavender	Lemon
Tea tree	Sweet orange
Thyme	Cardamom
Peppermint	Eucalyptus
Ginger	Roman chamomile

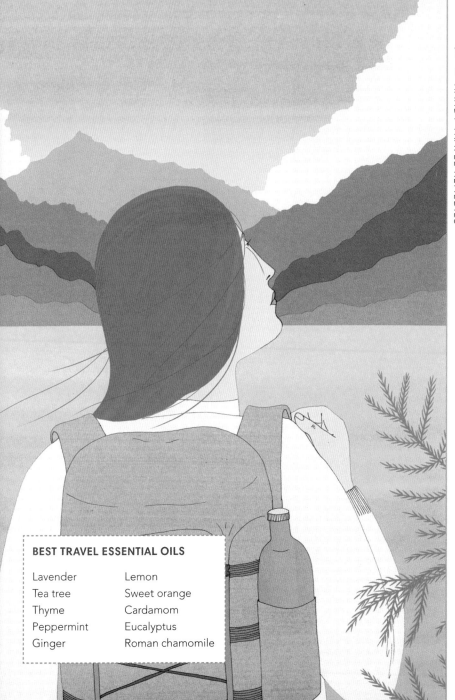

NATURAL ROOM REFRESHERS

Rather than use air fresheners full of artificial chemicals to scent your home, use essential oils to bring the scents of nature inside and infuse your home with the serenity of a spa.

Whatever the size of your living room or work space, diffusing essential oils can set the mood in a room, clear the air of germs, get rid of unwanted smells – or simply enhance your environment. Here are some combinations to help you wake reinvigorated, cleanse and enliven a sickroom, and keep your kitchen fresh. Once you are confident enough to create your own mixes, experiment with the oils suggested below. To get the most from a diffuser, keep doors shut to intensify the aroma and reap maximum rewards.

BEST ESSENTIAL OILS FOR ROOMS

Geranium	Clary sage
Sweet orange	Lavender
Lemon	Sweet marjoram
Grapefruit	Cardamom
Mandarin	Basil

BEDROOM WAKE-UP CALL

Get your day off to a great start with this lively, energizing blend of aromatic essential oils.

Makes 1 diffusion

Essential oils:

- 2 drops of cypress
- 2 drops of frankincense
- 2 drops of mandarin

Other items:

Room diffuser

How to make

Add the recommended amount of water to the diffuser, then add the drops of essential oils to the surface.

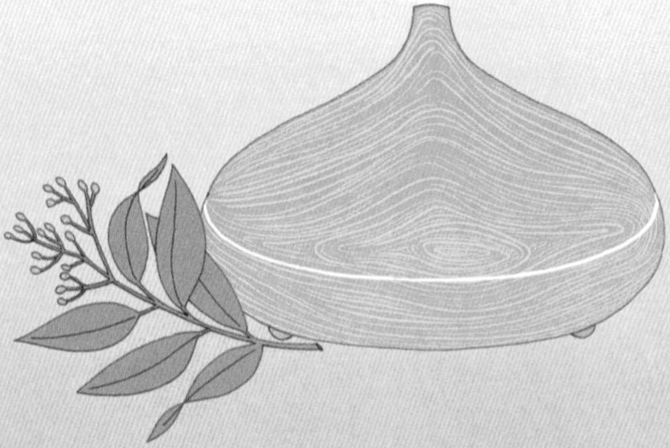

SICKROOM SOOTHER

This uplifting blend is made up of oils with antiviral, antibacterial, and antimicrobial properties to speed recovery.

Makes 1 diffusion

Essential oils:

- 2 drops of eucalyptus
- 3 drops of litsea
- 3 drops of ravensara

Other items:

Room diffuser

How to make

Add the recommended amount of water to the diffuser, then add the drops of essential oils to the surface.

KITCHEN ODOUR-BUSTER

Banish lingering cooking smells by spritzing your kitchen with this zesty and herby mix. Always spritz into the air and avoid spraying onto food.

Makes 1 spritz

Essential oils:

- 5 drops of eucalyptus
- 5 drops of lime
- 5 drops of rosemary

Other items:

Spray bottle

How to make

Fill the spray bottle with water and add the essential oils. Screw the nozzle on and shake to combine before every use.

ESSENTIAL OILS LIST

If the oils you buy do not have a botanical name in Latin on the label, or if the name does not match the Latin name listed, it may contain additives or be inauthentic. This list of the oils featured in this book also details the safety cautions you should take where necessary.

Achillea millefolium
YARROW
Avoid if pregnant, breast feeding, or if you have epilepsy.

Anthemis nobilis
ROMAN CHAMOMILE

Boswellia carterii
FRANKINCENSE

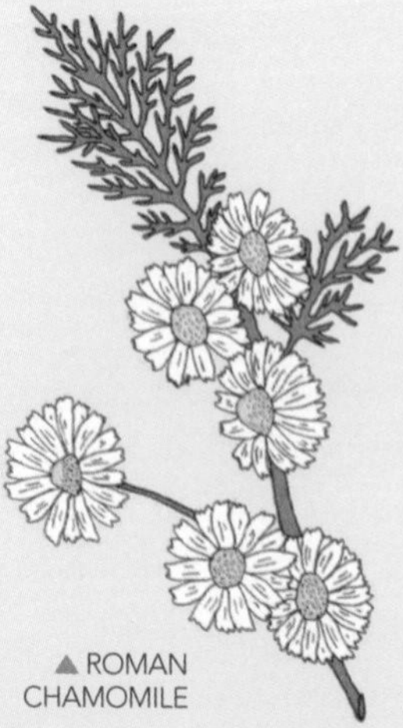

▲ ROMAN CHAMOMILE

Cananga odorata
YLANG YLANG
Can cause headaches if you are sensitive to strong odours.

Cedrus atlantica
CEDARWOOD ATLAS

Cinnamomum zeylanicum
CINNAMON LEAF
Avoid if pregnant; use in an under 1 per cent dilution (5 drops in 25ml) on sensitive skin.

Citrus aurantifolia
LIME
Only use lime essential oil marked as "Distilled" rather than "Expressed". Expressed lime essential oil can make the skin light-sensitive.

Citrus aurantium var. amara (flos)
NEROLI

Citrus aurantium var. amara (fol)
PETITGRAIN

Citrus bergamia
BERGAMOT
Only use if labelled "FCF Bergamot", otherwise it may make the skin light-sensitive. "FCF" means "furocoumarin free", and furocoumarins are a chemical compound in the plant that reduce the skin's ability to protect itself from the harmful effects of sunlight.

Citrus limonum
LEMON
Makes skin light-sensitive: use in an under 2 per cent dilution (6 drops in 15ml) if skin will be exposed to the sun within 12 hours of use.

Citrus nobilis/
Citrus reticulata
MANDARIN

Citrus paradisi
GRAPEFRUIT
Makes skin light-sensitive: use in an under 4 per cent dilution

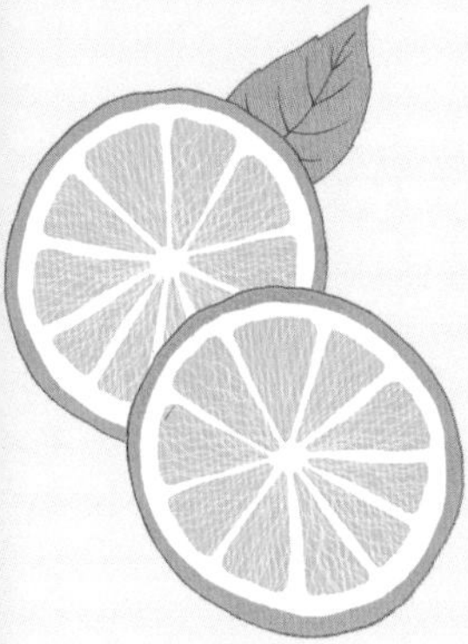

▲ SWEET ORANGE

(10 drops in 25ml) if skin will be exposed to the sun within 12 hours of use.

Citrus sinensis
SWEET ORANGE

Commiphora myrrha
MYRRH
If pregnant, use only in later stages of the third trimester, from no earlier than week 35.

Coriandrum sativum
CORIANDER

Cupressus sempervirens
CYPRESS

Cymbopogon citratus
LEMONGRASS
Use in an under 2 per cent dilution (6 drops in 15ml) on sensitive skin.

Cymbopogon martinii
PALMAROSA

Elettaria cardamomum
CARDAMOM

Eucalyptus citriodora
LEMON EUCALYPTUS

Eucalyptus globulus
EUCALYPTUS

Eucalyptus radiata
EUCALYPTUS RADIATA

Foeniculum vulgare var. dulce
SWEET FENNEL
Avoid if pregnant, or if you have oestrogen-dependent cancers; use in an under 2 per cent dilution (10 drops in 25ml) on sensitive skin.

Helichrysum italicum
IMMORTELLE

Jasminum officinale
JASMINE
If pregnant, use only in later stages of the third trimester, from no earlier than week 35.

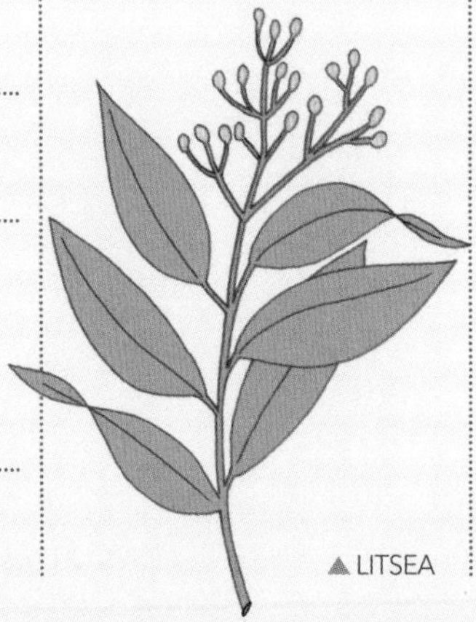

▲ LITSEA

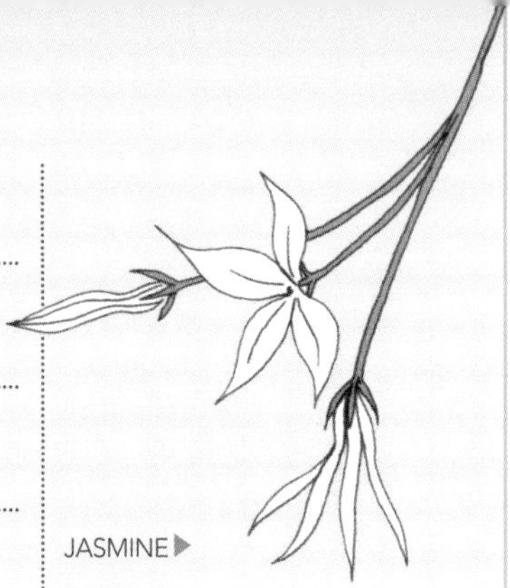

JASMINE ▶

Juniperus communis
JUNIPER

Laurus nobilis
BAY LAUREL
Avoid if pregnant, and do not use on sensitive skin. Use in an under 1.25 per cent dilution (6 drops in 25ml).

Lavandula angustifolia
LAVENDER

Lavandula x intermedia
LAVANDIN
Avoid if pregnant or epileptic.

Litsea cubeba
LITSEA
Use in an under 2 per cent dilution (6 drops in 15mls) on sensitive skin.

Matricaria recutita
GERMAN CHAMOMILE

Melaleuca alternifolia
TEA TREE

Melaleuca viridiflora
NIAOULI

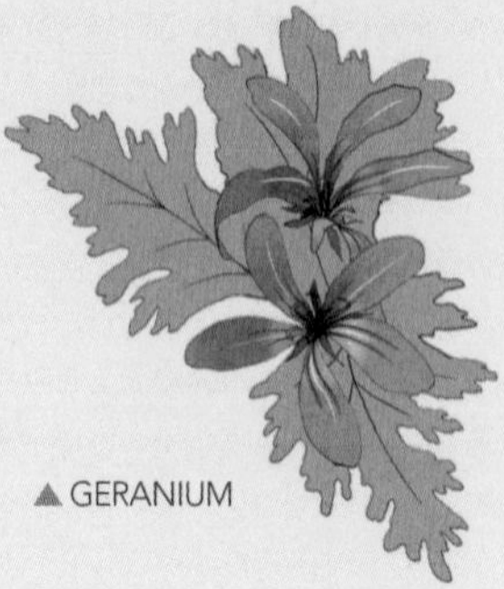

▲ GERANIUM

Melissa officinalis
MELISSA (LEMON BALM)
Use in an under 2 per cent dilution (6 drops in 15ml) on sensitive skin.

Mentha piperita
PEPPERMINT
Use in an under 1 per cent dilution (3 drops in 15ml) on sensitive skin.

Myrtus communis
MYRTLE

Ocimum basilicum CT linalool
BASIL
Avoid if pregnant. Use in an under 2 per cent dilution (6 drops in 15ml) on sensitive skin.

Origanum marjorana
SWEET MARJORAM

Pelargonium graveolens
GERANIUM

Picea mariana
BLACK SPRUCE

Pimpinella anisum
ANISEED
Avoid if pregnant, or if you have oestrogen-dependent cancers; use in an under 2.5 per cent dilution (5 drops in 10ml) on sensitive skin.

Pinus sylvestris
PINE
Use in an under 2 per cent dilution (6 drops in 15ml) on sensitive skin.

Piper cubeba
CUBEB

Piper nigrum
BLACK PEPPER

Pogostemon cablin
PATCHOULI

Ravensara aromatica
RAVENSARA

Rosa damascena
ROSE

Rosmarinus officinalis
ROSEMARY
Avoid if you have epilepsy.

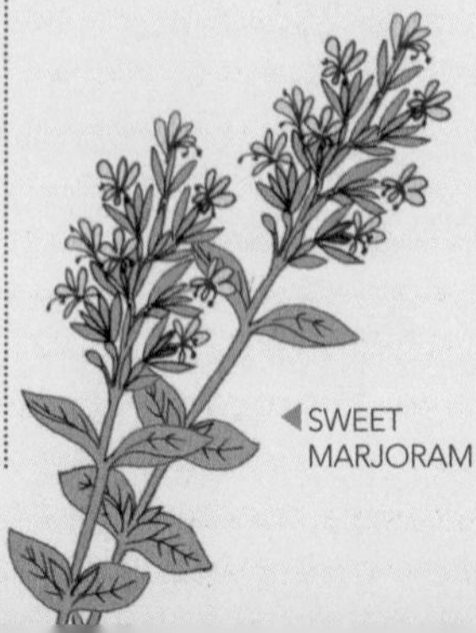

◀ SWEET MARJORAM

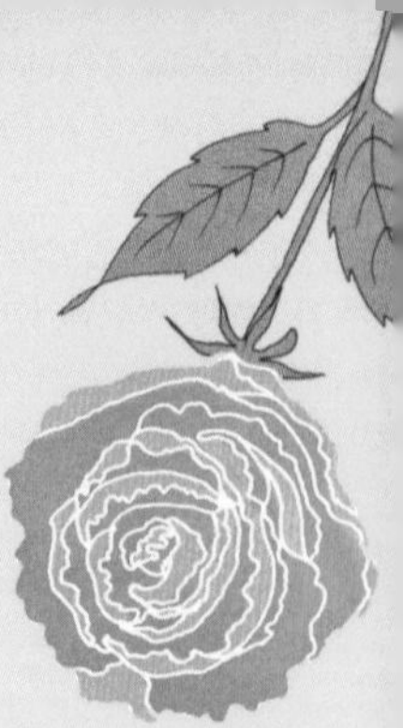

ROSE ▶

Salvia lavandulifolia
SPANISH SAGE
Avoid if pregnant, breast feeding, or if epileptic. Use in an under 2 per cent dilution (6 drops in 15ml).

Salvia sclarea
CLARY SAGE

Santalum album
SANDALWOOD

Thymus vulgaris CT linalool
THYME
Avoid the similarly-named *Thymus vulgaris CT thymol* if you have sensitive skin. It is high in phenol, an irritant.

Vetiveria zizanoides
VETIVER

Zingiber cassumunar
PLAI

Zingiber officinale
GINGER
If pregnant, use only in later stages of the third trimester, from no earlier than week 35.

RESOURCES

Aromatherapy is growing in popularity, and with so many practitioners springing up it's advisable to find a therapist through one of the internationally-recognized bodies detailed below. The suppliers listed are all well-respected and, in most cases, will ship their products worldwide.

FURTHER READING

Essential Oils Neal's Yard Remedies (DK)

Complete Massage Neal's Yard Remedies (DK)

Essential Oil Safety Robert Tisserand and Rodney Young (Elsevier)

SUPPLIERS OF ESSENTIAL OILS AND COMPLEMENTARY PRODUCTS

Neal's Yard Remedies www.nealsyardremedies.com

Penny Price Aromatherapy www.penny-price.com

Tisserand Aromatherapy www.tisserand.com

Oshadhi www.oshadhi.co.uk

Shechina Essential Oils www.shechina.co.uk

Base Formula www.baseformula.com

SOCIETIES, REGISTERS, AND AUTHOR'S WEB ADDRESS

The International Federation of Professional Aromatherapists (IFPA) www.ifparoma.org

The International Federation of Aromatherapists (IFA) www.ifaroma.org

The National Association of Holistic Aromatherapists (NAHA) www.naha.org

The Aromatherapy Trade Council (ATC) www.a-t-c.org.uk

Louise Robinson www.louiserobinson.co.uk

INDEX

Index entries in **bold** indicate specific wellbeing and healing practices.

M

N

O

ABOUT THE AUTHOR

Louise Robinson is a therapist with qualifications in aromatherapy, massage, and reflexology. She took up complementary therapy after 20 years in a successful corporate career. Having trained with Neal's Yard Remedies, she today runs a thriving therapy practice in Kent and works with the NHS mental health services within the Mother & Baby Unit at the Bethlem Royal Hospital. She is passionate about helping her clients through holistic therapeutic treatments, taking a combined approach where a person's physical and emotional conditions may be linked.

AUTHOR'S ACKNOWLEDGMENTS

Working on this book has been such a privilege and a joy for me, and it has been written with all of my wonderful clients in mind. I thank them for believing in me and for driving my passion to continually learn more and more about aromatherapy. To my teachers Victoria Plum and Elaine Tomkins, thank you for introducing me to the deeper therapeutic use of essential oils and the power of touch. You are both my constant inspiration as I continue on my journey as a therapist.

For your amazing support, guidance, encouragement, and patience, thank you Rona Skene, Ian Fitzgerald, Louise Brigenshaw, Dawn Henderson, Natalie Clay, and Kiron Gill at DK: you were all a joy to work with. Much thanks also to Harriet Lee-Merrion for the beautiful artworks that bring this book to life.

Thank you to all my friends for your love and encouragement. A special mention must go to my mentor and friend, Caroline Percy, for your unwavering support, encouragement, and your wise words!

Finally, and most of all, thank you to my wonderful family, my husband Cruz and sons Luke, Bode, and Adam for your constant love, backing, and faith in everything I do.

PUBLISHER'S ACKNOWLEDGMENTS

DK would like to thank the following for their assistance in the publication of this book: John Friend for proofreading, and Marie Lorimer for compiling the index.

DISCLAIMER

While the information in this book has been carefully researched, the publisher and authors are not engaged in providing health advice for individual readers. Neither the publisher nor the author can therefore accept any liability for loss, injury, or damage that is sustained by readers in consequence of adopting any suggestion or of using the information in this book.

If you have any health problems or medical conditions, consult with your physician before undertaking any of the exercises set out in this book. The information in this book cannot replace sound judgement and good decision-making when it comes to reducing the risk of injury, and you must take care.

Do not try to self-diagnose or self-treat serious or long-term problems without first consulting a qualified medical practitioner as appropriate. Always seek professional medical advice if problems persist. If taking prescribed medicines, seek medical advice before using any alternative therapy.

Do not use essential oils for conditions if you are undergoing a course of medical treatment, without seeking professional advice. Consult a qualified aromatherapist before using essential oils during pregnancy.